# OPML

OXFORD PAIN MANAGEMENT LIBRARY

# Acute Pain

# OPML

OXFORD PAIN MANAGEMENT LIBRARY

# Acute Pain

Edited by

## Lesley Bromley

Consultant in Anaesthesia,
University College London,
London, UK

## Brigitta Brandner

Head of Acute Pain Research Group,
University College London,
London, UK

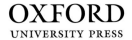

## OXFORD
UNIVERSITY PRESS

# OXFORD
## UNIVERSITY PRESS

Great Clarendon Street, Oxford OX2 6DP

Oxford University Press is a department of the University of Oxford.
It furthers the University's objective of excellence in research, scholarship,
and education by publishing worldwide in

Oxford New York

Auckland Cape Town Dar es Salaam Hong Kong Karachi
Kuala Lumpur Madrid Melbourne Mexico City Nairobi
New Delhi Shanghai Taipei Toronto

With offices in

Argentina Austria Brazil Chile Czech Republic France Greece
Guatemala Hungary Italy Japan Poland Portugal Singapore
South Korea Switzerland Thailand Turkey Ukraine Vietnam

Oxford is a registered trade mark of Oxford University Press
in the UK and in certain other countries

Published in the United States
by Oxford University Press Inc., New York

British Library Cataloguing in Publication Data

Data available

Library of Congress Cataloging in Publication Data

Data available

Typeset by Newgen Imaging Systems (P) Ltd., Chennai, India
Printed in Great Britain by Ashford Colour Press Ltd, Gosport, Hampshire
ISBN 978–0–19–923472–1

10 9 8 7 6 5 4 3 2 1

Whilst every effort has been made to ensure that the contents of this book are as
complete, accurate and-up-to-date as possible at the date of writing. Oxford
University Press is not able to give any guarantee or assurance that such is the case.
Readers are urged to take appropriately qualified medical advice in all cases. The
information in this book is intended to be useful to the general reader, but should
not be used as a means of self-diagnosis or for the prescription of medication.

# Contents

# Contributors

**Obi Agu**
Consultant Vascular &
Endovascular Surgeon,
University College Hospital,
London, UK

**Elizabeth Ashley**
Consultant in Anaesthesia,
University College London,
London, UK

**Sanjay Bajaj**
Pain Research Fellow,
University College London
Hospitals,
London, UK

**Brigitta Brandner**
Head of Acute Pain Research
Group,
University College London,
London, UK

**Lesley Bromley**
Consultant in Anaesthesia,
University College London

**Jeremy N. Cashman**
Consultant Anaesthesist,
St George's Hospital,
London, UK

**Sam Chong**
Department of Neurology,
King's College Hospital,
London, UK

**John F. R. Dick**
Consultant in Anaesthesia,
University College Hospital,
London, UK

**Mano Doriaswami**
Specialist Registrar in
Anaesthetics,
North Central London
School of Anaesthesia,
London, UK

**Johan Emmanuel**
Specialist Registrar in
Anaesthetics,
North Central London
School of Anaesthesia,
London, UK

**Shashi Gadgil**
Specialist Registrar,
Department of Geriatric
Medicine,
University College Hospital,
London, UK

**J. Ganesalingham**
Department of Neuroscience,
King's College Hospital,
London, UK

**Arif H. Ghazi**
Advanced Trainee in Pain
Management,
The Pain Management Center
National Hospital for Neu-
rology and Neurosurgery,
University College London
Hospitals Foundation Trust,
London, UK

**Upal Hossain**
Clinical Research Fellow in
Haematology,
Barts and the London NHS
Trust,
London, UK

**Richard Howard**
Consultant Anaesthesist,
The Hospital for Sick Children,
Great Ormond Street,
London, UK

**Damon Kamming**
Consultant Anaesthesist,
University College London,
London, UK

**Sue Mallett**
Academic Lead at RFH and
Head of Transfusion and
Coagulation Research Group,
Department of Anaesthesia,
Royal Free Hospital,
London, UK

**Anna L. Mandeville**
Consultant Clinical
Psychologist, Pain Management,
Psychological Medicine
Department,
London, UK

**Ali Mofeez**
Consultant in Anaesthesia and
Pain Management,
University College Hospital,
London, UK

**Ramini Moonsinghe**
Consultant Anaesthetist,
University College Hospital,
London, UK.

**James A. Smart**
Consultant in Anaesthesia,
University College Hospital,
London, UK

**Adrian Wagg**
Department of Geriatric
Medicine,
University College Hospital,
London, UK

**Suellen M. Walker**
Clinical Senior Lecturer in
Paediatric Anaesthesia and
Consultant in Paediatric
Anaesthesia and Pain
Medicine,
Portex Department of
Anaesthesia,
Institute of Child Health,
London, UK

**Edward Welechew**
Consultant in Anaesthesia
and Acute Pain Management,
Northern General Hospital,
Sheffield, UK

# Abbreviations

| | |
|---|---|
| AAA | abdominal aortic aneurysm |
| ATP | adenosine triphosphate |
| Bk | bradykinin |
| CB1 | cannabinoid receptor type 1 |
| CDH | chronic daily headache |
| CH | cluster headache |
| CL | clearance |
| CNS | central nervous system |
| COX | cyclooxygenase |
| CRPS | complex regional pain syndrome |
| CSF | cerebrospinal fluid |
| CT | computed tomography |
| CTG | cervicothoracic ganglion |
| GA | general anaesthesia |
| GABA | gamma aminobutyric acid |
| GBS | Guillain–Barré syndrome |
| GCA | giant cell arteritis |
| GCSF | granulocyte colony-stimulating factor |
| GFR | glomerular filtration rate |
| GI | gastrointestinal |
| Hb | haemoglobin |
| HIV | human immunodeficiency virus |
| IASP | International Association of the Study of Pain |
| in-PCA | intranasal PCA |
| LA | local anaesthesia |
| LFTs | liver function tests |
| M3G | morphine-3-glucuronide |
| M6G | morphine-6-glucuronide |
| MMT | methadone for maintenance therapy |
| MOH | medication overuse headache |
| MRI | magnetic resonance imaging |

| MRI | magnetic resonance imaging |
|------|------|
| NCA | nurse-controlled analgesia |
| NGF | nerve growth factor |
| NHS | National Health Service |
| NICE | National Institute for Clinical Excellance |
| NNT | number-needed-to-treat |
| NRS | numerical rating scale |
| NSAIDs | non-steroidal anti-inflammatory drugs |
| PAC | preassessment clinic |
| PADSS | post-anaesthetic discharge scoring system |
| PAG | periaqueductal grey |
| PAN | primary afferent nociceptor |
| PCA | patient-controlled analgesia |
| PCB | para cervical block |
| PCEA | epidural PCA |
| PH | paroxysmal hemicrania |
| PHN | postherpetic neuralgia |
| PONV | post-operative anti-inflammatory drugs |
| SCD | sickle cell disease |
| Sc-PCA | subcutaneous PCA |
| TAO | thromboangitis obliterans |
| TCAs | tricyclic antidepressants |
| TENS | transcutaneous electrical nerve stimulation |
| TRPV1 | transient receptor potential vanilloid 1 |
| TTH | tension-type headache |
| VAS | visual analogue scale |
| VD | volume of distribution |
| VRS | verbal rating scale |

# Chapter 1

# The physiology of acute pain

Lesley Bromley

### Key points

- Acute pain as a result of tissue damage is self-limiting.
- Impulses are generated in primary sensory nerves by chemical mediators released from the damaged tissues.
- The spinal cord receives these impulses in the dorsal horn.
- At the level of the spinal cord, the impulses can be amplified or reduced in amplitude by descending inputs.
- At the level of the spinal cord, the representation of the painful area and the sensitivity of other, surrounding areas can be modified.
- At the level of the brainstem and thalamus, further modification can take place.
- The final perception of the pain can be modified by other central phenomena such as anxiety and fear.
- New imaging techniques have allowed a greater understanding of cortical representation of pain.
- The role of the glia in maintaining painful states is evolving.

## 1.1 Introduction

Our understanding of the physiology of acute pain has grown enormously in the past 50 years. This is a result of an increase in the understanding of how the nervous system detects painful stimuli, and how it then processes the information. Since the time of the earliest anatomists, it was evident that the nervous system conducted information to the brain. Philosophers such as Descartes thought that the nerves 'opened up pores in the common sense centre'. We now know that the old idea of nerves as a form of wiring is too simplistic and that the nervous system is essentially a plastic system, which is capable of modifying the information that arrives at the brain at every synapse along the way.

Pain is a sensation that requires an intact nervous system and an intact consciousness to interpret the incoming stimuli. It is a complex construct, influenced by many factors both physiological and psychological. The physiological transmission of nociceptive impulses requires the interpretation of those signals by the conscious brain as pain. The understanding of the transmission processes has evolved somewhat faster than our understanding of the processing and interpretation undertaken by the cortex. Melzack (1999) has written about the body-self neuromatrix, which receives inputs from many aspects of physiology and combined with psychological elements results in an output called pain (see Figure 1.1). In this chapter, the current understanding of the nociceptive pathways will be discussed, with some reference to emerging understanding about central processing.

## 1.2 Nociception pathways

### 1.2.1 The periphery

Tissue injury causes the disruption of cells and the release of their contents into the interstitial space. A number of responses and reflexes occur. The inflammatory response is initiated, drawing in white cells and mast cells that release histamine. The resulting mixture of chemicals released from damaged cells and inflammatory mediators has been referred to as the sensitizing soup. The contents of the soup bind to receptors on the primary afferent nociceptor (PAN) (Table 1.1).

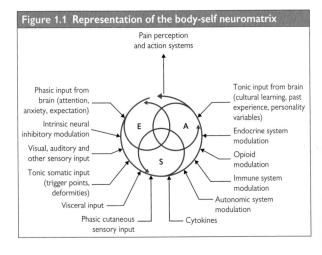

**Figure 1.1 Representation of the body-self neuromatrix**

Pain perception and action systems

Phasic input from brain (attention, anxiety, expectation)

Intrinsic neural inhibitory modulation

Visual, auditory and other sensory input

Tonic somatic input (trigger points, deformities)

Visceral input

Phasic cutaneous sensory input

Cytokines

Tonic input from brain (cultural learning, past experience, personality variables)

Endocrine system modulation

Opioid modulation

Immune system modulation

Autonomic system modulation

| Table 1.1 Sensitizing soup |
| --- |
| • Prostaglandins |
| • Bradykinins |
| • 5-HT |
| • Na+ |
| • $K^+$ |
| • $H^+$ |
| • Adenosine triphosphate |
| • Histamine |
| • Nerve growth factor |

PANs are C-fibres, lying in the tissues, with their cell bodies in the dorsal route ganglia of the spinal cord, and dendrites extending into the laminae of the dorsal horn of the cord. They terminate in laminae I and II, the outer part of lamina II receives exclusively C-fibre input. They express many receptors on their surfaces and are listed in Table 1.2.

When these receptors are activated, by binding the elements of the sensitizing soup, there is a lowering of the firing threshold of the nerve. The nerve then fires and action potentials travel to the spinal cord.

Increased levels of firing in the PAN may be accompanied by firing of large $A\delta$ fibres. These conduct so-called fast pain, which is described as sharp or pricking pain, whereas C-fibre-mediated pain is described as burning and aching pain. $A\delta$ fibres are myelinated and have faster conduction velocities than C-fibres, they project to lamina I and to laminae III and IV of the dorsal horn.

There are three distinct routes by which the nociceptor is stimulated. In the first case, protons that are in higher concentration as the pH of the tissue falls during injury, act at the transient receptor potential vanilloid 1 (TRPV1) receptors.

Second, direct binding to the appropriate receptor by the inflammatory mediators, for example, bradykinin (BK), to BK-1 and BK-2 receptors, which alter sodium ion conductance, serotonin to $5\text{-HT}_{2A}$ receptors, and nerve growth factor (NGF), which binds to TrKA receptors. Adenosine triphosphate released from damaged cells acts both directly by binding to receptors and indirectly by releasing adenosine, which binds to $A_2$ receptors. $P_2X_3$ receptor is a purine receptor associated with acute nociceptive transmission. Glutamate, acting on both AMPA and NMDA receptors, also has a role in peripheral sensitization.

Third, indirect mechanisms, many inflammatory cells also express TrkA receptors; therefore, the release of NGF stimulates these cells

| Table 1.2 Receptors on the primary afferent neurone |
|---|
| • Vanilloid receptor/TRPV1 receptor |
| • Sensory neurone specific (SNS) sodium channel |
| • NGF receptors |
| • BK receptors |
| • CB1 receptors |
| • $P_2X_3$ purine receptors |
| • Voltage-gated calcium channels |
| • TrkA receptors |
| • Glutamate receptors |
| • Adenosine $A_2$ |

to release more 5-HT and histamine. Arachidonic acid metabolites, prostaglandins, and leucotrienes may also increase the release of 5-HT and histamine, potentiate currents through the sensory-specific sodium channels, and enhance currents through TRPV1 channels. As inflammation continues, sympathetic terminals release prostaglandins under the influence of BK.

### 1.2.2 **The dorsal horn**

Impulses in the PAN pass into the dorsal horn of the spinal cord. The dorsal horn acts as an integrating centre. The primary impulse can be modified in several ways before it is passed up to the cortex.

Perhaps the best known of these modifications was set out in the Gate theory proposed by Melzack and Wall (1965). They showed that input from other neurones to the dorsal horn, principally low-threshold myelinated fibres, could reduce the onward nociceptive traffic passing up to the brain. This theory, proposed in the 1960s, started a new way of thinking about pain transmission, and in the 1980s Wall and Woolf suggested that rather than a simple gate, the response to primary nociceptive input was in fact highly variable, and the system was plastic (can change shape), the theory of neuroplasticity (Cook *et al* 1987).

#### 1.2.2.1 *Central sensitization and wind up*

Incoming impulses in the primary afferent reach the synapse in between the primary and secondary afferents at different layers of the dorsal horn (see Figure 1.2). The primary afferent releases glutamate and substance P. These transmitters are released into the cleft and bind to receptors on the secondary afferent. This has two effects; there is a spatial and temporal alteration in the sensitivity of local secondary afferents. This results in areas around the damaged tissue, which are intact, showing hyperalgesia and allodynia.

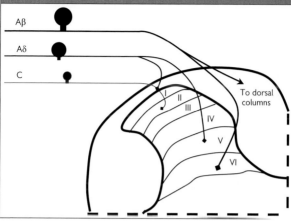

**Figure 1.2 Primary sensory neurone termination in the dorsal horn**

Aβ

Aδ

C

I
II
III
IV
V
VI

To dorsal columns

Glutamate binds to two receptors on the secondary afferent, NMDA and AMPA. During the initial phase, glutamate binds to AMPA, and incoming traffic in the primary nerve matches outgoing traffic in the secondary nerve. When a threshold of AMPA activity is reached, conformational changes occur which allow NMDA to bind glutamate. As soon as this occurs, the traffic in the secondary afferent rises dramatically and exceeds the incoming traffic (see Figure 1.3). This is wind up.

#### 1.2.2.2 *Descending inhibition*

Pathways descend from higher centres to interact at the synapse of the primary and secondary afferents. The descending signal, derived from the cortex, hypothalamus, and amygdala, is integrated in the periaqueductal grey (PAG) matter in the brainstem. It then passes downwards to the dorsal horn. The whole of this pathway is very rich in opiate receptors. In addition, 5-HT and adrenaline are expressed as transmitters in this system. The adrenergic expression in this pathway is thought to explain the phenomena of battle field analgesia, where soldiers with terrible injuries report no pain whilst in the field.

Other inhibitory systems in the dorsal horn include a $\alpha_4\beta_2$ nicotinic acetylcholine receptor, which is specific for human antinociception, and cannabinoid receptor type 1 (CB1).

### 1.2.3 **Ascending to higher centres**

The final integrated signal travels up the spinal cord in the lateral spinothalamic tracts. Information is integrated in the brainstem, the

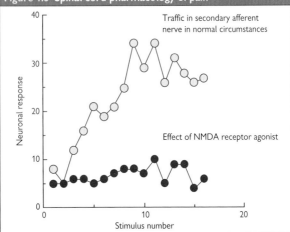

**Figure 1.3 Spinal cord pharmacology of pain**

Traffic in secondary afferent nerve in normal circumstances

Effect of NMDA receptor agonist

Neuronal response

Stimulus number

PAG, the medulla, and the rostral pons. Projections from this area go to the thalamus. Thalamus is another site of integration of signals, but also has an interesting role in generating signals and projections to higher centres, which can occur without input from the spinal cord. This is the phenomenon sometimes seen with brainstem strokes of thalamic pain.

The use of functional magnetic resonance imaging has allowed a better understanding of the function of higher centres in pain perception. The concept of a pain centre, such as Descartes described, has been superceded, and the current concept is of a pain matrix. This is composed of thalamus, the primary and secondary sensory cortex, the insula cortex, the anterior cingulate cortex, and motor regions including the cerebellum. Feeding into this matrix are contributions from the limbic system, particularly associated with the effect of emotional state on pain perception, and many levels of the central nervous system (CNS) seem to contribute to the effect of distraction on pain perception. Reported pain is less during tasks that require concentration, and the more complex the task the lower the reported pain.

Recent studies have shown that the insular cortex, which is deep in the cortical structure, has a somatic representation of pain in a manner similar to the sensory cortex, and it seems to provide the affective component of pain. Along with the cingulate cortex the insular is responsible for signalling the unpleasantness of pain, whereas the sensory cortex seems to be responsible for the simple sensory component of pain.

In rodents, the most frequently studied species, there are distinct gender differences in pain responses. Male mice express NMDA receptors with higher thresholds than female mice. Central processing of pain also has gender differences. Patterns of responses in the pain matrix seem to vary according to the gender. There is some evidence that this may be true in humans. The menstrual cycle may be the significant factor, as animal evidence suggests that the expression of receptors and the turnover of receptors in membranes are both influenced by the hormonal milieu.

## 1.3 The role of the glia

The physiology of pain has been elucidated with regard to neurons, their networks and pathways. The glial cells of the CNS have been considered until very recently to provide nothing more than a physical structure or framework to support the neurons. Glial cells express all the receptors that neurones express and their cytoplasm contains all the enzymes of the arachidonic acid pathway. It would seem likely therefore that the cells would be, at a very minimum, altered in some way by the incoming nociceptive impulses. The role of the glia is probably more pronounced in persistent pain rather than in acute tissue injury. A protein named HIV-1gp120, which accumulates in the cerebrospinal fluid (CSF) of HIV positive patients, has been shown to activate glial cells and produce an exaggerated pain state via nitric oxide pathways. Activated glia cells release cytokines into the CSF and these then act to lower conduction thresholds in nociceptors, and can produce spontaneous firing of nociceptors, NGF. Interleukin-1$\beta$ (IL-1$\beta$) and tumour necrosis factor-$\alpha$ are implicated. IL-10, an inhibitory cytokine, given by infusion has been shown to attenuate the effects of these pro-inflammatory cytokines. Intrathecal IL-10 has been shown to attenuate neuropathic nerve injury pain in rats, and plasmid encoding for IL-10 given to rats, raised levels of native IL-10, and reduced pain behaviour in nerve constriction injury.

## 1.4 The future

The expanding knowledge of the physiology of nociception and pain processing, combined with the psychological understanding of the human perception and behavioural response to pain, adds to the complexity of the process. Complexity is a useful characteristic as it also increases the potential for intervention. The large number of receptors involved in nociceptive transmission and the multiple synapses, both in the peripheral nervous system and in the CNS, make it quite obvious that effective pain management is not going to involve a single drug or intervention. A multimodal approach to altering pain physiology and perception is the way forwards. Acute pain is normally self-limiting. As healing occurs, mediator levels drop in the peripheral tissue and the system returns to its baseline state. Some patients go on to have persistent pain despite healing, and the mechanisms that turn an acute pain episode into a persistent pain state are not clear. The underlying mechanisms for this transition from acute to persistent pain would be of great value, and establishment of the role of acute pain management in the prevention of this transition is a significant area of research for the future.

## References

Casey KL (2000). Concepts of pain mechanisms: the contribution of functional imaging of the human brain. *Progress in Brain Research*, **129**, 277–87.

Clark A, Gentry C, Bradbury E, McMahon S, and Malcangio M (2007). Role of spinal microglia in rat models of peripheral nerve injury and inflammation. *European Journal of Pain*, **11**, 223–30.

Cook AJ, Woolf CJ, Wall PD, McMahon SB (1987). Dynamic receptive field plasticity in rat spinal cord dorsal horn following C-primary afferent input. *Nature*, **325**, 151–3.

Dickenson AH (1995). Spinal cord pharmacology of pain. *British Journal of Anaesthesia*, **75**, 193–200.

Fields HL and Basbaum AI (1999). Central nervous system mechanisms of pain modulation. In Wall PD and Melzac R, eds. *Textbook of pain*, 4th edn, p. 309–29. Churchill Livingstone, Edinburgh.

Melzack R (1999). From the gate to the neuromatrix. *Pain*, **S6**, S121–6.

Melzack R and Wall PD (1965). Pain mechanisms: a new theory. *Science*, **150**, 971–9.

Richardson JD and Vasko MR (2002). Cellular mechanisms of neurogenic inflammation. *Journal of Pharmacology and Experimental Therapeutics*, **302**, 839–45.

# Chapter 2

# The pharmacology of the drugs used in acute pain

Lesley Bromley

> ## Key points
>
> - Drug treatment is the mainstay of acute pain management.
> - An understanding of the pharmacology of the drugs used is essential for rational acute pain management.
> - Drugs that have a primary analgesic action have been used traditionally.
> - Recently, adjunct drugs and combinations have been shown to be more effective than analgesics alone.
> - In the past 20 years, the route of administration and the timing of analgesic drugs have played a greater part in efficient acute pain management.

## 2.1 Drugs with a primary analgesic action

### 2.1.1 Opioid drugs

Opioid drugs are those having an agonist action at opioid receptors. The original drugs in this class were derived from opium, a naturally occurring plant extract, but many are now chemically synthesized. Conventionally, drugs derived from natural sources acting at opioid receptors are called opiates. Those synthesized chemically are called opioids.

#### 2.1.1.1 *Opioid receptors*

All drugs in this class have their action by binding with opioid receptors. These receptors have now been cloned and mammalian opioid receptors are now known to be of four types: OP1, OP2, OP3, and ORL1. The relationship of this new classification with the former system is shown in Table 2.1.

Each receptor type has a naturally occurring ligand, the peptides that bind to opioid receptors OP1–OP3 are collectively called endorphins

| Table 2.1 Opioid receptors | |
|---|---|
| Ligand-based classification | Structural classification |
| δ-Receptor | OP1 |
| κ-Receptor | OP2 |
| μ-Receptor | OP3 |
| Orphan receptor | ORL1 |

and consist of three different groups, the enkephalins, endomorphins, and dynorphins. The fourth group of receptors, the ORL1 group, was identified in 1997, and the ligand was later identified as orphanin FQ. This receptor and its ligand have a central role in response to stress and an analgesic role in the dorsal horn of the spinal cord.

Opiate receptors are G-protein receptors linked to a potassium channel. Binding of an agonist produces two effects in the cell:

- An influx of potassium, causing hyperpolarization of the postsynaptic cell
- A reduction in cyclic AMP in the presynaptic cell.

G-protein receptors have multiple binding sites, and can be modified by the occupation of intracellular binding. The opioid receptor varies in its sensitivity to agonists and is influenced by the amount of cholecystokinin expressed in the cell.

Opioid receptors are subject to ligand-directed trafficking. In this process, the ligand receptor complex is rapidly internalized and removed from the receptor population, this occurs only with certain agonists (e.g. fentanyl), and it is not seen with morphine.

The exact state of activity of the opioid receptors is therefore a complex interaction, including the following:

- States of phosphorylation of the G protein
- Interactions with other intracellular mediators
- The temporal relationship of stimulation by ligands.

All interact to set and reset the sensitivity of the receptor. This complexity, only partially understood, explains why individuals can have very different pharmacological responses to opioid drugs.

### 2.1.2 **Opioid analgesic drugs in common use**

All drugs act at the OP3 receptor to produce analgesia.

Drugs vary in their potency at the OP3 receptor, and this may influence their use. While increasing the intensity of the analgesia produced, this will also increase the unwanted effects such as respiratory depression.

In summary, it is the pharmacokinetic differences between the drugs that account for different clinical usage.

### 2.1.2.1 *Morphine, diamorphine, and codeine*

Morphine and codeine are extracted from raw opium, and this remains the most economical means of production. They are the most commonly used opiates.

Diamorphine is semi-synthetic, and is a prodrug with no direct action on OP3 receptors. It is hydrolysed by tissue esterases to 6-monoacetylmorphine, and then to morphine. Diamorphine is pharmacodynamically identical to morphine.

All three drugs can be given orally, but the bioavailability is variable, 25–50% for morphine and 50% for codeine. When diamorphine is given orally, no diamorphine can be detected in the systemic circulation, as it is rapidly metabolized by enzymes in the gut wall and liver; however, as the metabolites are active it has a significant pharmacodynamic effect. Diamorphine has poor stability in solution, and is presented as a powder for reconstitution. Once dissolved it has a shelf-life of 48hr, which has discouraged its oral use.

Morphine is metabolized to morphine-6-glucuronide and morphine-3-glucuronide, the former is active at the OP3 receptor. Both metabolites are excreted in the urine.

Codeine metabolism is by demethylation to morphine. There is genetic variability in this process, codeine is a prodrug that undergoes hepatic metabolism to morphine. The cytochrome enzyme CYP2D6 catalyses the conversion. There are more than 50 genetic variants of this enzyme, 20% of the population are poor metabolizers of codeine and will therefore experience little analgesia when given the drug. Thus, when codeine is used, it is important to monitor the individual to ensure that a pharmacological effect is achieved.

### 2.1.2.2 *Pethidine*

Pethidine is a synthetic opioid, less potent than morphine, but at equipotent doses causes the same side effects. Respiratory depression will occur with pethidine if large doses are given.

It is orally active with a bioavailability of 50%. It has a short duration of action than morphine with a half-life of 3–4hr. It has two unique properties, that is, it has membrane-stabilizing properties and shows weak local anaesthetic action on peripheral nerves. It has marked anticholinergic properties related to its chemical structure. It is metabolized to norpethidine, which can cause central excitation and convulsions. Long-term administration of high doses is required to produce significant amounts of norpethidine.

### 2.1.2.3 *Fentanyl, alfentanil, sufentanil, and remifentanil*

These four drugs are chemically related.

*Fentanyl*, the parent drug, is 100 times more potent than morphine at the OP3 receptor. This family of drugs has been developed for use in anaesthesia, and they share the common features of high lipid solubility, short duration of action, and high potency at OP3.

They are all given intravenously for use in anaesthesia. Fentanyl has been formulated in a transbuccal lozenge that can be used for breakthrough pain and as a transdermal patch, which can be used for acute and chronic pain management. The lozenge is rapid in onset (5–15mins) and has an elimination half-life of 3.5hr. It is metabolized in the liver to inactive metabolites.

*Alfentanil* is less potent than fentanyl at the OP3 receptor. It has a shorter half-life than fentanyl because, being less lipid soluble, it has a smaller volume of distribution. It is a highly basic compound, and at plasma pH 89% of the drug is unionized producing a large concentration gradient for the drug into the central nervous system (CNS). It is metabolized to inactive metabolites. Alfentanil is frequently given by infusion because of its short half-life. However, it is cumulative given over long periods, and its context-sensitive half-life increases with duration of infusion.

*Sufentanil* is the most potent of this family of drugs, being 600–800 times more potent than morphine. It is used extensively in anaesthesia, and has been used in very small doses for intravenous patient-controlled analgesia (PCA). However, it has never been available in the United Kingdom, and because of the profound respiratory depression it produces, it is difficult to use safely in intravenous PCA.

*Remifentanil* has approximately the same potency as fentanyl. It has a unique method of metabolism, the molecule contains an ester bond that can be acted upon by plasma esterases and therefore it has a very short half-life not dependent on liver function. This makes it a very suitable drug for delivery by infusion during general anaesthesia. It is not licensed for use as an analgesic in conscious spontaneously ventilating patients unless an anaesthetist is in direct supervision. However, a number of case reports have been published where remifentanil has been used by low dose continuous infusion for the relief of labour pain to good effect.

### 2.1.2.4 *Oxycodone*

Oxycodone is a semi-synthetic opioid, which has been available alone or in combination with paracetamol in the United States for some 40 years. It is available in an immediate release form for use in post-operative and other acute pain. The oral immediate release form has a rapid onset of action 10–15min with a peak effect in 30min to 1hr. It is 45% protein bound and has a half-life of 2–3hr. It is metabolized in the liver by the same enzyme system as codeine, CYP2D6, and as a result there is genetic variation in response to the drug. It has two weakly active metabolites. In acute pain, oral doses of 5–10mg of immediate release oxycodone are equivalent to 10mg of intramuscular morphine. The slow release preparation is available in doses of up to 120mg and has been used in the management of chronic pain. Large dose of slow release oxycodone should not be given to patients who are naive to opiates. In the United States, there has been much concern about the abuse potential of these large doses of oxycodone, which seems to be the equivalent of morphine.

Oxycodone can cause all the side effects that other opiates produce, but is said to produce less itching and less nausea.

### 2.1.2.5 *Methadone*

Methadone was first synthesized 60 years ago. It is pharmacodynamically indistinguishable from morphine, but it has a high oral bioavailability, its action is terminated by redistribution and it is cumulative. Its elimination half-life is long between 20hr and 45hr. It has some action at the NMDA receptor which may add to its analgesic properties.

## 2.1.3 **Non-steroidal anti-inflammatory drugs**

This group of drugs inhibits the action of the enzyme cyclooxygenase (COX). This enzyme catalyses the production of prostaglandins and thromboxanes from the compound arachidonic acid. The enzyme exists in several isoforms: COX-1 is the so-called constitutive isoform that takes part in the regulation of platelet and renal function, and maintains the integrum of the gastric mucosa; COX-2 is the inducible form, the production of which is upregulated in inflammatory processes; and COX-3 is a variant of COX-1 and has a key role in the CNS.

The early non-steroidal anti-inflammatory drugs (NSAIDs) were non-selective in their enzyme blockade, producing analgesia but also unwanted effects on the renal, platelet, and gastric mucosal function. Research to produce a more selective COX-2 inhibitor was intended to produce a drug that provided analgesia without the effect on the constitutive enzyme. A series of drugs with a range of selectivity were introduced under the banner of COX-2 inhibitors, early optimism for these drugs was dashed by the realization that in chronic use in patients with rheumatoid and osteoarthritis they produced a significant excess cardiac mortality. In some cases, it would appear that even short-term use could produce a higher incidence of cardiac events. We are therefore left with the non-selective drugs in our pharmacopoeia.

### 2.1.3.1 *Diclofenac*

Diclofenac is chemically an acetic acid derivative. It has an oral bioavailability of 60% due to first pass metabolism in the liver. Its elimination half-life is 1–2hr and it is 99.5% protein bound. It is formulated for the oral, rectal, topical, and parenteral routes. It is also presented in an oral form as a slow release formulation to extend its action.

If analgesic efficacy is expressed in a number of patients, who need to receive the drug for one patient to have a 50% reduction of pain (number-needed-to-treat, NNT), then diclofenac, 100mg, has an NNT of 1.9. However, it does not provide sufficient analgesia on its own to treat pain in the first hours post-operatively, but if given with opioids it has been shown to reduce the requirements for opioids, the so-called opioid sparing effect.

### 2.1.3.2 *Ketorolac*

Ketorolac is also an acetic acid derivative and is indicated specifically for the treatment of post-operative pain. It is a racemic mixture of S- and R-isomers, of which the S-isomer is active. It has an elimination half-life of 4–10hr and is 99% protein bound.

It has been implicated in acute renal failure in the post-operative period, related to hypovolaemia during surgery.

Ketorolac, 30mg intramuscularly, has an NNT of 3.4, which indicates that it is less effective than diclofenac.

### 2.1.3.3 *Dexketoprofen*

The proprionic acid derivatives are all presented as racaemic mixtures of D and S isomers. Dexketoprofen is the S(+) enantiomer of ketoprofen, which has all the analgesic activity. The R(−) enantiomer is inactive. It has the same bioavailablility of ketoprofen, but is more rapidly absorbed, and has a more rapid onset of action. It is completely metabolized in the liver to inactive metabolites. It is unselective for COX enzyme. It is available as an oral preparation and in a parenteral form. It is effective as an analgesic and has been used extensively in dental and post-operative pain. It has NNTs of 3 for the 25mg dose and 2.1 for the 50mg dose. In common with all NSAIDS it has an opiate sparing effect in acute postoperative pain, its rapid onset makes it useful in acute pain.

### 2.1.3.4 *The proprionic acid derivatives: ibuprofen, ketoprofen, naproxen, and fenoprofen*

This group of NSAIDs are all used as oral preparations. They typically have a good oral bioavailability; ibuprofen 78%, high protein binding, around 99%, and low clearance. They are non-selective, but have relatively lower potency both for analgesia and unwanted effects. Ibuprofen 400mg orally has an NNT of 2.4.

### 2.1.3.5 *The oxicams*

*Piroxicam* has a high oral bioavailability and has an elimination half-life of over 50hr. It is also 99% protein bound. Piroxicam 20mg has an NNT of 2.7.

*Tenoxicam* is also well absorbed orally and has an even longer half-life of 72hr.

### 2.1.3.6 *Paracetamol*

Paracetamol is not classified as an NSAID, it has no perpheral COX blocking activity, but has weak activity against central COX-3 enzyme.

This is probably not the primary mechanism that produces its analgesic effect. The mechanism of analgesic action of paracetamol has been recently elucidated. Paracetamol acts as a prodrug in the CNS. It is deacylated to *p*-aminophenol and in turn conjugated with arachidonic acid to form *N*-arachidonoyl-phenolamine. This compound is an endogenous cannabinoid, acting at CB1 receptors, and is also an agonist at TRPV1 receptors.

It is well absorbed orally with an 85% oral bioavailability, 20% is protein bound, specifically to albumin. It is metabolized in the liver and conjugated with glucuronide (60%), sulphide (35%), and cysteine (3%). In excessive doses, N-hydroxylation produces an intermediary compound of high reactivity, which is deactivated by reaction with glutathione. When glutathione becomes depleted, the N-hydroxylated intermediary reacts with hepatic proteins causing hepatic necrosis.

Paracetamol is not sufficiently potent to produce adequate analgesia in moderate to severe pain, 1000mg orally has an NNT of 4.6, that is, one out of every five patients with moderate to severe pain would get a 50% reduction of pain intensity who would not have done so with placebo.

Combination preparations of paracetamol and weak opiates have been used. Paracetamol plus codeine 60mg adds an extra 11% response. Paracetamol combination with dextropropoxyphene was withdrawn in January 2005 because of concerns over overdose and toxicity.

Paracetamol is available as oral, rectal, and intravenous preparations.

### 2.1.4 Tramadol

Tramadol is a synthetic, centrally acting analgesic, it is a racemic mixture of two stereoisomers. Its mode of action has two elements. It is a weak OP3 agonist, 6000-fold less binding than morphine. It also increases the central neuronal synaptic levels of 5-hydroxytryptamine and noradrenaline by preventing their reuptake. These two effects are supra additive for analgesia, but are additive or counteractive for the adverse effects.

It has a good oral bioavailability, and a half-life of 7hr. It is metabolized by CYP2D6 enzymes to *O*-desmethyltramadol. This metabolite has a higher affinity for OP3 receptors than the parent compound.

### 2.1.5 Buprenorphine

Buprenorphine is a semi-synthetic, highly lipid-soluble opioid derived from thebaine. It is 20 times more potent than morphine 0.4mg being equivalent to 10mg of morphine. It is a partial agonist at the OP3 receptor with which it binds and slowly dissociates. It has a slower onset of opiate type side effects, but they are more difficult to reverse with naloxone due to the binding affinity of the drug.

It is well absorbed especially sublingually with a rapid onset and peak effect within 2hr. Its half-life in the plasma is 3hr, but its avid binding means that effects last much longer than predicted by the half-life. It is 96% protein bound. Most of the drug is excreted unchanged.

As with all opioids, side effects are common, and nausea and vomiting are said to be more common with buprenorphine.

## 2.2 Local anaesthetic agents

Local anaesthetic agents are used to block sensory nerves and thereby reduce nociceptive input to the nervous system. This produces analgesia, but also reduces all sensory inputs so that the area blocked will be numb, and insensitive to hot and cold as well. Local anaesthetics are used to produce analgesia via a number of routes, including local infiltration, nerve blocks, and spinal and epidural instillation.

Local anaesthetics block sodium channels in the neurone, preventing the conduction of action potentials and thus block all traffic in the neurone. As sensory neurones travel in mixed nerves, there may be an element of motor blockade produced.

Local anaesthetic agents pass through the cell membrane and ionize inside the cell, entering the sodium channel from its interior aspect to bind and block the passage of sodium. Nociception is conducted in C-fibres and Aδ-fibres. The former are small diameter, unmyelinated and are therefore more sensitive to local anaesthetic penetration.

### 2.2.1 Lidocaine

An amide local anaesthetic, therefore heat stable, lidocaine is commonly used for local anaesthesia because of its rapid onset, 2–5min and relatively short duration of action 1–2hr. In terms of analgesia, it is useful to establish a block rapidly, but because of its short duration the requirements to 'top up' or reapply the drug are both inconvenient and can lead to a phenomenon known as tachyphylaxis. In tachyphylaxis, increasing doses of the drug are required to produce a given effect. All local anaesthetics are subject to this but it is most marked with lidocaine.

### 2.2.2 Bupivacaine

Bupivacaine is also an amide local anaesthetic, but has a slower onset of action approximately 20min, and a longer duration of action up to 5hr. This drug is commonly used for epidural and spinal analgesia.

Bupivacaine toxicity is related to its affinity for sodium channels, particularly in the heart. This is true of all local anaesthetic agents, but bupivacaine is particularly difficult to displace from the channel making resuscitation difficult. The drug is a racemic mixture of two isomers, and the S-enantiomer is marketed as levobupivacaine and is said to have less toxicity.

### 2.2.3 Ropivacaine

This drug was developed to produce a drug with similar length of action of bupivacaine without the motor block and cardiotoxicity. While it has a wider therapeutical index and seems to be less likely to produce ventricular fibrillation, the separation of sensory and motor block is more difficult to demonstrate.

## 2.3 Non-traditional drugs and cannabinoids

### 2.3.1 Ketamine

Ketamine is an NMDA receptor antagonist.

Ketamine has complex actions at the opioid receptors, has a local anaesthetic action, acts at muscarinic and nicotinic receptors, and can reduce calcium influx through voltage-sensitive calcium channels. Because of this complex pharmacology, all involving receptor systems that are known to be involved in spinal cord transmission, it is difficult to identify exactly what the role of the NMDA receptor interaction is in the analgesia produced by ketamine.

In human volunteers, ketamine reduces the magnitude of both primary and secondary hyperalgesia after a burn injury. Perhaps, the most important question with regard to post-operative pain is the contribution made to the experience of post-operative pain by the secondary hyperalgesia and wind up phenomena. Intravenous ketamine has been shown to be additive to intravenous opiates when given as a single bolus dose per-operatively. Stubhaug et al. (1997) demonstrated that the use of continuous intravenous ketamine reduced PCA consumption of morphine for the first few hours post-operatively; thereafter, there was no difference. They also mapped the punctate hyperalgesia around the wound and demonstrated that the area of central sensitization was greatly reduced compared with placebo. This was not related to a reduction in pain scores or of analgesia consumption. Ketamine does reduce secondary hyperalgesia and allodynia around a surgical wound, the extent to which this reduces pain scores is not clear. Ketamine does have a role in managing patients who are accelerating their use of opiates with no increase in analgesia. A one-off ketamine infusion can reduce the opiate requirements in these patients.

### 2.3.2 Gabapentin

Gabapentin is a drug that was introduced for the management of chronic pain and is finding a role in the management of acute pain.

The mechanism of action of gabapentin has been established as binding to the $\alpha_2\delta$ subunit of the presynaptic voltage-gated calcium channel in spinal nociceptive neurones. Binding results in the inhibition of calcium influx and a commensurate reduction in the release of excitatory transmitters in the pain pathway. Its relative pregabalin has a better pharmacokinetic profile.

Studies have shown that premedication with gabapentin reduces post-operative analgesia use and reported pain. However, it is not licensed for this use. The increasing body of evidence from the literature supports the use of gabapentin and more studies using pregabalin are awaited. The optimal premedication dose is not yet clearly established.

### 2.3.3 **Cannabinoids**

While no preparations of cannabinoids are available for acute pain at the present time in the United Kingdom, there have been a number of trials looking at the efficacy of various cannabis-related preparations.

Canpop®, a combination of tetrahydrocannabinol and cannabidiol, in the ratio of 1:0.5 has been studied and shown to have analgesic action. Canpop® (10mg) had an NNT of 2 and 15mg had an NNT of 1.3, and this should be compared with tramadol 100mg with an NNT of 2.4. However, the higher dose did produce a large number of unwanted effects including lightheadedness and euphoria.

## References

Dickenson AH (2002). Gate control theory of pain stands the test of time. *British Journal of Anaesthesia*, **88**(6), 755–7.

Gregg A, Francis S, Sharpe P, and Robotham D (2001). Analgesic effect of gabapentin premedication in laparoscopic cholecystectomy: a randomised double blind placebo controlled trials. *British Journal of Anaesthesia*, **87**, 174P (abstract).

Holdcroft A, Maze M, Doré C, Tebbs S, and Thompson S (2006). A multicenter dose-escalation study of the analgesic and adverse effects of an oral cannabis extract (Cannador) for postoperative pain management. *Anesthesiology*, **104**, 1040–6.

Medge D and Owen MD (2002). Prolonged intravenous remifentanil infusion for labor analgesia. *Anesthesia & Analgesia*, **94**, 918–19.

Seib R and Paul J (2006). Preoperative gabapentin for postoperative analgesia: a meta-analysis. *Canadian Journal of Anaesthesia*, **53**, 461–9.

Stubhaug A, Brevik H, Eide PK, Kreunen M, and Foss A (1997). Mapping of punctate hyperalgesia around a surgical incision demonstrates that Ketamine is a powerful suppressor of central sensitisation to pain following surgery. *Acta Anaesthesiologica Scandinavica*, **41**, 1124–32.

Williams DG, Patel A, and Howard R (2002). Pharmacogenetics of codeine metabolism in an urban population of children and its implications for analgesic reliability. *British Journal of Anaesthesia*, **89**, 839–45.

Yaksh TL (1997). Pharmacology and mechanisms of opioid analgesic activity. *Acta Anaesthesiologica Scandinavica*, **41**, 94–111.

# Chapter 3

# Non-pharmacological methods of acute pain management

Anna L. Mandeville

## Key points

- Psychological factors are a key part of pain perception as articulated in the neuromatrix model of pain.
- Psychoeducational interventions are of significant value in acute pain management and have reduced pain severity, distress, and length of hospital stay.
- Mood, beliefs about pain and illness, previous experience of pain, and the behaviour of health care professionals all influence pain perception and response to pain.
- Helping patients reappraise the threat value of pain through tailored information giving and where needed cognitive behavioural interventions are practical strategies.
- Attention control methods, including clinical hypnosis, are effective in reducing procedural pain.

## 3.1 Neuropsychology of pain

The neuromatrix model of pain (Melzack 1999) recognizes the key contributions made by central nervous system processing to the pain experience. Ascending peripheral inputs combine with descending neural pathways in a plastic, recursive system, and modulate transmission from the first synapse onwards. Cortical processing including beliefs, experience, fears, and mood are powerful descending influences.

Psychological factors can then exert control over sensory input (Melzack & Wall 1965) and are therefore pivotal in the management of all pain, acute or chronic. This has been well demonstrated in experimental and clinical settings.

## 3.2 **Context of acute pain**

### 3.2.1 **Medical and surgical patients**

Moderate to severe acute pain is commonly experienced by medical or surgical patients and this may continue after initial discharge (Bruster *et al* 1994). The inpatient population has so far been the focus of the majority of research into acute pain, where it is the most common cause of delayed discharge from hospital.

### 3.2.2 **Acute pain in the community**

Patients also consult about acute pain in the community setting, for example, in the presentation of nociceptive pain (musculoskeletal and visceral pain) in primary care. Acute pain can also become persistent for a proportion of patients. Therefore, acute and chronic pain should not ultimately be thought of as disparate entities, but as a potential continuum.

## 3.3 **Psychological predictors of pain intensity and persistence**

### 3.3.1 **Medical and surgical patients**

Preoperative anxiety or low mood have been associated with higher post-surgical pain intensity in a range of procedures including abdominal, bypass, and knee surgeries (e.g. Kalkman *et al* 2003). Patients' underlying thoughts or 'cognitions' about their condition and its potential consequences, or the treatment they are receiving, may provoke or maintain anxiety and low mood. The lack of control in hospital environments and poor communication from health care professionals may exacerbate this (Salmon 2000). Fearful beliefs and thoughts may be followed by behaviours that appear uncooperative, such as non-adherence to mobilization, through fear of increasing pain or causing damage.

A thinking style that has been particularly associated with anxiety and mood disturbance is termed 'catastrophizing'. This is described as a process whereby individuals overestimate the threat value of a situation and underestimate the resources they have to bring to bear on the challenge. This produces excessively fearful thoughts, which then provoke distress. Catastrophizing has been found to be predictive of higher pain intensity, following a range of surgical interventions (Sullivan *et al* 2001). Whether it is situationally specific or an individual trait is not clear (Turner *et al* 2001).

### 3.3.2 **Community patients**

Psychological factors in the context of non-surgical acute pain are also risk factors for the development of persistent pain, for example, in musculoskeletal conditions. Similar to acute pain in an inpatient setting, these also include low mood, a catastrophic thinking style, negative expectations about pain, and avoidance of activities that are feared may exacerbate pain (Vlaeyen & Linton 2000).

## 3.4 Psychological interventions in acute pain

A meta-analysis of 191 studies (Devine et al 1992) provides some broad evidence that psychosocial interventions in inpatient surgical settings can have a beneficial effect on recovery, reducing pain intensity, distress, and length of hospital stay compared with placebo or care as usual. This analysis included a wide range of approaches, such as providing information, encouraging questions, teaching skills such as reappraising thoughts, relaxation exercises, or hypnosis. These approaches are further considered later in the chapter.

### 3.4.1 Role of information giving in acute pain

Although it makes intuitive sense, information giving is not as straightforward as it appears. It is easy to assume all information is benign, but this may not be the case. Some patients habitually cope by *avoiding* detailed information, for example, about medical or surgical procedures (procedural information) or what the sensory experience may involve (sensory information) (Salmon 2000). Clinicians can 'screen' for whether patients would like more or less detailed information in a simplistic manner, by asking patients whether or not they would like to know more.

For patients who generally welcome information, combining procedural and sensory information (telling the patient what will happen and how it may feel) has been shown to reduce acute pain and distress during various diagnostic, medical, and dental procedures. This may be through an enhanced sense of control or trust in the clinician. The combination is still effective with regard to surgical procedures, but less so.

Surgical patients seem to benefit from procedural rather than sensory information, although these benefits decline as surgery becomes more major, where perhaps the information is more inherently distressing (Australian and New Zealand College of Anaesthetists 2005). All information giving is enhanced by a sensitive communication style, where patients have the opportunity to ask questions. It is also maximized by being given in the context of an ongoing relationship with a caregiver, rather than coming from multiple clinicians who have little idea with regard to a patient's ongoing concerns.

Patients with acute musculoskeletal pain also present to general practitioners (GPs) in the community. These patients may also benefit from early information and exploration of concerns. Advice for acute back pain sufferers is to keep as active as possible. Some patients are at risk of increasing the chances of their pain becoming chronic, perhaps through fears of re-injury on activity. These patients are then likely to get into a cycle of increasing disability as they reduce their activities in the mistaken belief that this is protective against future pain (Vlaeyen and Linton 2000). Patients may well respond to exploration of worries and encouragement in resuming normal activity. Those whose pain does not resolve at 6–8 weeks may need more intensive support to identify barriers in more detail, set goals, and work towards goals (Von Korff and Moore 2001).

### 3.4.2 Eliciting patients' concerns

Clinicians often assume that patients will be helped by 're-assurance', but patients told that 'they don't need to worry' may be discouraged from asking questions they feel they need answers to. Patients' concerns may appear idiosyncratic to health professionals but are often driven by personal experience or misinterpretations.

> **Box 3.1 Patients' concerns are driven by personal experience or misperceptions**
>
> Beliefs about medications
> *'I am resistant to medicines. If they give me a normal anaesthetic I know I will wake up in the middle of the operation. The pain will kill me'*
>
> Extrapolating from family experience
> *'My uncle had this same operation and died'*
>
> Misinterpretation of body sensations
> *'I can feel the stitches tearing every time I move'*

22

### 3.4.3 Helping patients re-appraise their thoughts and beliefs

Being able to elicit and listen to patient's beliefs and expectations is an important intervention in acute pain settings. As we have seen alarmist thinking styles are associated with increased pain and distress and finding out and discussing fears opens the possibility of helping patients re-appraise misperceptions or exaggerated beliefs and thoughts. This may well leave them feeling less threatened by procedures and more able to feel they can meet the challenge of treatments. In turn this may reduce pain and distress or help them to adhere to treatment plans.

### 3.4.4 Attentional control

The direction of attention away from an acute pain stimulus (distraction) is commonly employed by health care professionals. Consider, for example, the GP asking a patient about holiday plans whilst administering an injection or taking a blood sample. Other manipulations of attention are more formal and can be very effective in acute pain, particularly procedural pain.

## Box 3.2 Helping patients to re-evaluate

Patients are generally helped to re-think their conclusions and beliefs by being encouraged to gently challenge them through further reflection. Direct confrontation may leave patients more confrontation

| Thought/belief | Helpful questions to challenge thoughts | Well meant but less helpful response |
| --- | --- | --- |
| 'I am resistant to medicine. I know I will wake up in the middle of the operation. The pain will kill me' | How likely do you think this is?<br>Do you know about how anaesthetists assess and monitor patients?<br>Would it be helpful to know more? | 'That's not going to happen in this hospital'<br>'That's really rare and you don't need to worry about it' |
| 'My uncle had this same operation and died' | I'm sorry to hear that. You must be frightened! Do you know what happened?<br>What would make you feel easier about having the procedure, given this is your experience?<br>Are there particular questions you would like to ask? | 'That won't happen to you, don't worry'<br>'Only a small proportion of people die during this operation, so its not really worth thinking about' |
| 'I can feel the stitches tearing every time I move' | That sounds like a horrible feeling! What makes you think its definitely the stitches?<br>Has anyone explained the kinds of feelings you can get in your body after this sort of operation | 'It's not the stitches. They don't tear like that'<br>'You're worrying too much. The stitches are really strong' |

Hypnosis can be used in a variety of ways to redirect attention in relationship to acute pain. Internal distraction (e.g. focussing on imagined stimuli such as pleasant scenes or memories) may be used. Alternatively, the focus may be directed towards external stimuli, such as images projected on to a wall, or listening and becoming very involved with the hypnotist's voice. These techniques are generally thought to absorb the patient in alternative stimuli to the pain. The mechanism of pain reduction is not completely clear, but is not opiate or relaxation dependent. The process may encourage descending inhibition (see Box 3.1) or temporarily block the patient's subjective awareness of the pain sensation. Magnetic resonance imaging studies have also shown that a reduction in anterior cingulate cortex activity correlates with reported changes in sensory-affective reports from patients in hypnosis (Rainville 1997).

Within hypnosis, suggestions may also be given to change the intensity of a sensation or relabel it, for example, changing a sharp pain to a tingling sensation. More ambitiously, full hypnotic anaesthesia can be suggested, so that a body part is experienced as completely numb. Full hypnotic anaesthesia is quite hard to achieve and more possible on subjects who are highly hypnotizable and probably highly practised. Some training in hypnosis is needed, but it is a skill which is potentially accessible to health care professionals and can augment existing skills. One meta-analysis yielded effect sizes of 0.64–0.74 in the use of clinical hypnosis to reduce acute pain in a range of clinical and experimental settings (Montgomery 2000), suggesting training may well be worth the investment.

### 3.4.5 **Enhancing a sense of control and resourcefulness**

As reviewed above, spending time eliciting patient's thoughts and beliefs and helping them to re-evaluate them where necessary or helpful is a key intervention that can arguably be employed by most health care professionals, as can working sensitively with patients' needs for information (Box 3.2). This is probably sufficient for most patients who also draw on networks of personal support including family, friends, and other patients.

For highly distressed patients, perhaps those who are finding it difficult to progress with rehabilitation or those struggling to feel confident to return home from hospital, more intensive intervention may be needed in the form of more specialist psychological support. This may come from the growing body of Clinical Health Psychologists specifically employed in pain management or in medical settings to help teams integrate psychological care more closely into their work.

A clinical psychologist will use psychological interventions such as cognitive behaviour therapy to help patients challenge 'catastrophic thoughts' in more detail, or help them to activate their own problem-solving abilities. They may also help medical teams with any interaction or communication problems that have arisen.

## References

Australian and New Zealand College of Anaesthetists and Faculty of Pain Medicine (2005) *Acute Pain Management Scientific Evidence*; 2nd Edition.

Bruster S, Jarman B, Bosanquet N, Weston D, Erens R al (1994) National survey of hospital patients. *BMJ*. **309**. 1542–6.804.

Devine EC. (1992) Effects of psychoeducational care for adult surgical patients: a meta-analysis of 191 studies. *Patient Educ Couns*, **19**,129–42.

Kalkman CJ, Visser K, Moen J, Bonsel GJ, Grobbee DE, Moons KG (2003). Preoperative prediction of severe postoperative pain. Pain, **105**, 415–23.

Melzack, R. (1999). From the gate to the neuromatrix. *Pain*, **Suppl 6**, 121–6.

Melzack R, Wall PD. (1965) 'Pain Mechanisms: A New Theory' in Pain: A Handbook for Nurses, Sofaer, B. (1984) Harper & Row, London.

Montgomery GH, David D, Winkel G, Siverstein JH, Bovbjerg DH. (2002). The effectiveness of adjunctive hypnosis with surgical patients: A meta-analysis. *Anesthesia and Analgesia*, **94(6)**, 1639–45.

Rainville P, Duncan GH, Price DD, Carrier B, Bushnell MC (1997) Pain affect encoded in human anterior cingulate but not somatosensory cortex. *Science*, **Aug 15;277(5328)**, 968–71.

Salmon P (2000) *Psychology of medicine and surgery*. London: Wiley.

Sullivan, MJ; Thorn, B; Haythornthwaite, JA; Keefe, F; Martin, M; Bradley, LA; Lefebvre, JC.(2001) Theoretical perspectives on the relation between catastrophizing and pain. *Clin J Pain*, **17**, 52–64.

Turner JA, Manci L, Aaron LA (2004) Pain-related catastrophizing: a daily process study. *Pain*, **110(1–2)**, 103–11.

Vlaeyen JW and Linton SJ. (2000). Fear-avoidance and its consequences in chronic musculoskeletal pain: A state of the art. *Pain*, **85**, 317–32.

Von Korff M and Moore JE. (2001) Stepped care for back pain: Activating approaches for primary care. *Annals of Internal Medicine*, **134**, 911–17.

# Chapter 4

# Acute pain management in principle

Jeremy N. Cashman

> ### Key points
>
> - Pain measurement is essential in evaluating response to analgesic therapy.
> - The oral route is the route of choice for analgesics in non-fasting patients.
> - Administering opioids by the neuraxial route provides superior analgesia to the same drug administered by parenteral routes.
> - Clinical practice guidelines may be useful in acute pain management.
> - Acute Pain Services improve the quality of post-operative pain management.

According to the International Association for the Study of Pain, acute pain is the pain of recent onset and probable limited duration which usually has an identifiable temporal and causal relationship to injury or disease. Acute pain is common, particularly in the post-operative period. However, acute pain may be due to non-surgical as well as surgical causes and affects patients in the community as well as patients in hospital. Consequently, although this chapter will focus on the management of acute post-operative pain, the basic principles will be applicable to other acutely painful conditions.

## 4.1 Assessment of acute pain

Assessment of acute pain is essential for the establishment of effective pain treatment.

Key factors in assessment include establishing the underlying cause and extent of injury or disease; characterizing and quantifying the pain; and selecting appropriate therapy and evaluating the response to therapy. Commonly, post-operative pain (whether somatic or visceral in origin) is nociceptive, is correlated with the operation site, is predictable, and is transient. However, occasionally neuropathic pain may also be present (Table 4.1).

### 4.1.1 **Pain measurement**

Pain measurement is a specific aspect of pain assessment which aims to quantify pain in order that the response to therapy can be evaluated. Acute nociceptive pain is more commonly assessed using single dimension pain scales than multidimensional pain scales (which can be useful for assessing neuropathic pain). Single dimension tools tend to measure pain intensity only whereas multidimensional tools assess the sensory, affective, and evaluative components of pain. Any measure of pain should be reliable, valid, and sensitive to change. Nevertheless, it is not the measurement tool itself but the performance of assessment that is important. Table 4.2 details some of the commonly used tools.

#### 4.1.1.1 *Categorical scales*

The simplest subjective measure of pain is to ask the patient whether or not s/he feels any pain. Greater sensitivity is obtained if ordered categories are used to grade the pain. A four-descriptor verbal rating scale (VRS; None–Mild–Moderate–Severe) is most commonly used, often with a numerical score allocated to a descriptor. Increasing the number of categories increases sensitivity, namely

0—No pain
1—Mild pain on movement only
2—Mild pain at rest and/or moderate pain on movement
3—Moderate pain at rest and/or severe pain on movement
4—Severe pain at rest and/or unbearable pain on movement
5—Unbearable pain

| Table 4.1 Features suggestive of neuropathic pain |
| --- |
| • History consistent with nerve injury |
| • Pain within but not necessarily confined to an area of sensory deficit |
| • Pain without evidence of ongoing tissue damage |
| • Pain burning, pulsing, shooting, or stabbing in character |
| • Paroxysmal or spontaneous pain |
| • Associated dysaesthesias |
| • Allodynia, secondary hyperalgesia, hyperpathia |
| • Associated autonomic features |

| Table 4.2 Instruments for pain assessment | |
| --- | --- |
| Unidimensional | Verbal rating scale (VRS) |
| | Numerical rating scale (NRS) |
| | Visual analogue scale (VAS) |
| | Picture scales |
| Multidimensional | McGill pain questionnaire (MPQ) |
| Others | Analgesic requirement |
| | Global scales |
| | Surveys |

Categorical scales are quick and simple to use. Furthermore, the verbal descriptors may reflect some of the multidimensional nature of pain. However, the scale cannot be assumed to be ordinal as intervals between word categories do not necessarily represent identical steps in pain intensity.

### 4.1.1.2 *Numerical scales*

Alternatively, the patient may be asked to give their pain a numerical score out of ten where 0 is no pain and 10 is the worst pain imaginable (numerical rating scale, NRS). NRS may be verbal or written. The NRS, similar to the VRS, is also quick and simple to use but is more sensitive than the VRS. The verbal NRS is the most commonly used bedside pain assessment tool.

When using the visual analogue scale (VAS) to measure pain intensity, the patient is asked to mark on a 10cm line with the ends labelled 'no pain' and 'worst pain imaginable' the point corresponding to their pain. The pain rating is obtained by measuring the distance in millimetres between 'no pain' and the 'patient's mark'. A rating <45mm is indicative of 'mild pain', 45–74mm is indicative of 'moderate pain', and >70mm is indicative of 'severe pain'. The VAS is a more sensitive indicator of pain intensity than other single dimension pain scales. In addition, it accurately represents changes in pain intensity but up to a quarter of patients may be unable to use it.

### 4.1.1.3 *Pictorial scales*

Pictorial scales are particularly useful for measuring pain in children. A series of faces (usually five or six) depicting a range of expression from tearfulness to happiness are shown to the child who is asked to point to the face that most closely mirrors how they feel. A numerical score is allocated to each face. Parents and carers can also use this tool.

### 4.1.1.4 *Multidimensional tools*

Multidimensional tools require patients to identify those descriptors from a series of word lists that accurately characterize their pain. Such scales represent the affective and evaluative components of pain as well as pain intensity but can be cumbersome to apply in the post-operative setting.

### 4.1.1.5 *Other tools*

The requirement for analgesics, for example, as recorded by a patient-controlled analgesia (PCA) machines, can be used as a surrogate measure of pain. Global scales tend to measure overall effectiveness of treatment and as such are more appropriate for outcome evaluation. Finally, the Department of Health requires hospitals to obtain feedback from patients about their experiences of, rather than satisfaction with care, including pain experience. Such surveys provide pain experience.

## 4.2 **Delivery of drugs**

The US Food and Drug Administration recognizes 111 distinct routes for drug administration. However, only a proportion of these routes are appropriate for systemic analgesic drug administration (Table 4.3).

### 4.2.1 **Enteral**

#### 4.2.1.1 *Oral*

The oral route is the most commonly used route of drug administration overall and is the route of choice in the non-fasting patient. However, the delay between drug administration and onset of effect is at least 20min, and is often much longer. Speed of absorption depends on whether tablets, capsules, suspension, enteric coating, sustained, or slow release preparations are used. In addition, presystemic metabolism can markedly reduced bioavailability of some drugs (e.g. morphine). Thus, the potency ratio of oral to parenteral morphine is 1:6 for acute pain. Systematic reviews have confirmed the effectiveness of preoperative oral coxibs and post-operative immediate release oral opioids for post-surgical pain. Controlled release oral opioids should not be used as sole agents for early post-surgical pain relief.

#### 4.2.1.2 *Rectal*

The rectal route is useful when other routes cannot be used. Rectal administration minimizes the likelihood of presystemic metabolism but correct placement of the suppository is important; too high inside the rectum results in absorption into the superior rectal vein resulting in greater first pass metabolism. Even with correct placement drug absorption can be very variable. Similarly, absorption is more variable and bioavailability is decreased by suppository insertion into a colostomy. In general, rectal opioid dosing roughly equates to oral opioid dosing, that is, potency ratio 1:1 with similar duration of effect.

| Table 4.3 Routes of systemic drug administration | |
|---|---|
| Enteral | Oral |
| | Rectal |
| Parenteral by injection | Intramuscular |
| | Subcutaneous |
| | Intravenous |
| Parenteral other than by injection | Transdermal |
| | Transmucosal |
| | Inhalational |
| Neuraxial | Epidural |
| | Intrathecal |
| Other | Intra-articular |
| | Intra-wound |

### 4.2.2 **Parenteral by injection**

#### 4.2.2.1 *Intramuscular*

The simplicity of this route means that it is probably the most commonly used route of analgesic drug administration post-operatively. However, absorption can be variable with respect to speed of onset, intensity and duration of analgesia, and repeat needling is often necessary. Insertion of an indwelling cannula, for example, into the deltoid muscle, circumvents this problem. Injection should be into a well-perfused muscle. A single 10mg intramuscular injection of morphine is effective in the initial treatment of moderate to severe post-operative pain with number-needed-to-treat (NNT; the number of patients needed to be treated for one patient to experience at least 50% pain relief) of 2.9 compared with placebo.

#### 4.2.2.2 *Subcutaneous*

This route of administration is popular for continuous infusion in non-acute pain management. Concentrated (hence small volume) aqueous, non-irritating solutions should be used and the infusion site should be changed regularly. Absorption can be unpredictable. Subcutaneous and intramuscular drug administration regimens can be used interchangeably.

#### 4.2.2.3 *Intravenous*

The 'gold standard' because of rapidity of onset and because it avoids uncertainty of drug absorption. However, the plasma level of drug declines rapidly, resulting in short-lived analgesia. This problem can be overcome by titrating a predetermined dose of opioid intravenously at fixed time intervals until pain is relieved (e.g. morphine 2–3mg bolus at 5min dose intervals), followed by a continuous opioid infusion after a further time interval. Alternatively, intravenous PCA (the on-demand, intermittent, self-administration of an analgesic drug by the patient) can provide effective analgesia whilst allowing for wide interpatient variation. Subcutaneous (sc-PCA), epidural (PCEA), and intranasal (in-PCA) routes can also be used. Intravenous PCA is more effective than conventional administration of opioid analgesics with no increase in opioid-related side effects whilst subcutaneous PCA is as effective as intravenous PCA.

### 4.2.3 **Parenteral other than by injection**

#### 4.2.3.1 *Transdermal*

Transdermal drug delivery allows for controlled release of drug with avoidance of first pass metabolism but drug uptake is influenced by skin blood flow. Although there are many topical non-steroidal anti-inflammatory drug (NSAID) preparations, there is no evidence for significant benefit of topical over oral NSAID in the treatment of minor non-surgical pain. Highly lipophilic opioids are ideally suited to transdermal drug delivery. With the early opioid patches, drug delivery rate was dependent on a rate-controlling membrane; thus, the area of applied patch determined the dose. With the newer transdermal therapeutic matrix systems, there is no drug reservoir or rate-controlling membrane as the opioid is dissolved in the adhesive matrix itself. Wash-in and washout of drug is therefore faster. Nevertheless, passive transdermal fentanyl administration is not currently recommended for post-operative pain relief. However, active transdermal fentanyl administration using iontophoresis (electrically charged molecules of ionized drug propelled through the skin by an external electrical field) shows promise as a method of PCA.

### 4.2.3.2 *Transmucosal and intranasal*

Buccal, sublingual, and intranasal routes of administration provide direct drug entry into the systemic circulation with avoidance of the problems of presystemic metabolism and are unaffected by the delay in gastric emptying that occurs during the perioperative period. Swallowing of drug will reduce efficacy. Sublingual buprenorphine and buccal fentanyl have been shown to be effective after abdominal surgery. Although several opioids have also been shown to be effective intranasally, including patient-controlled intranasal diamorphine, there are insufficient data at the present time to support the routine use of intranasal analgesia for acute post-operative pain.

### 4.2.3.3 *Inhalational*

Although clinical data exists for the effectiveness of nebulized analgesic drug administration, the data are insufficient at the present time to support the use of this route for acute post-operative pain.

## 4.2.4 **Neuraxial**

### 4.2.4.1 *Epidural*

Analgesic drugs may be administered into the epidural space as intermittent injection, continuous infusion, or even as PCEA (a lockout time of 10–20min is recommended, as is a basal infusion). In the case of lipid-soluble opioids such as fentanyl, the injection site should be 'dermatome specific'. Administering opioids by the epidural route provides analgesia that is superior to the same drug given as a continuous intravenous infusion and is associated with a reduced overall incidence of pulmonary complications. However, the incidence of transient neuropathy is 1:6000 whilst that of permanent neurological damage varies between 1:2000 and 1:20000. The incidence of epidural haematoma varies between 1:10000 and 1:100000 whilst the incidence of epidural abscess with prolonged epidural catheterization is 1:4500.

### 4.2.4.2 *Intrathecal*

Direct injection of opioid into the cerebrospinal fluid is associated with potent segmental analgesia using much smaller doses of opioid (commonly one-fifth) than that required for epidural analgesia. Onset is also faster than the epidural route. Otherwise, the same considerations apply.

### 4.2.5 Other

#### 4.2.5.1 *Intra-articular*

Intra-articular injection of morphine following knee joint arthroscopy can reduce post-operative pain for up to 24hr.

#### 4.2.5.2 *Intra-wound*

Studies of wound infiltration in post-operative pain are inconclusive.

## 4.3 Organization and objectives of Acute Pain Services

The earliest report of a structured approach to the management of post-operative pain with a ward-base epidural analgesia service appeared in 1988. In 1990, a joint report of the Royal Colleges of Surgeons and of Anaesthetists advocated the creation of an organized multidisciplinary acute pain team in all major hospitals. This concept has been widely adopted, not just in the United Kingdom, but throughout the world. Currently, over 85% of hospitals in the United Kingdom and North America have an established Acute Pain Service with dedicated pain nurses, and consultant sessions in acute pain.

### 4.3.1 Structure of an Acute Pain Service

The provision of safe and effective acute pain management is the ultimate goal of an Acute Pain Service but how the service is organized to deliver this goal varies widely. Nevertheless, there are several essential elements of an effective Acute Pain Service and these are outlined in Table 4.4.

A number of different personnel may be involved in an Acute Pain Service including anaesthetists, nurses, surgeons, pharmacists, physiotherapists, and even clinical psychologists. There are two different formats for Acute Pain Services. The service may be nurse-led by a clinical nurse specialist with varying degrees of anaesthetist supervision

| Table 4.4 Essential elements of an Acute Pain Service |
| --- |
| • Personnel |
| • Service delivery |
| • Assessment |
| • Analgesia |
| • Monitoring |
| • Documentation |
| • Education |
| • Audit and research |

progressing through to the anaesthetist as leader of a comprehensive multidisciplinary team. These two formats represent the opposite ends of a spectrum and most services fall somewhere in the middle. In the United Kingdom, 95% of Acute Pain Services are consultant-led and 5% are nurse-led. Furthermore, the spectrum of activity may vary from supervision of primarily specialized techniques of pain relief to involvement in all forms of pain management for all patients within an institution (except obstetrical patients who are generally managed by a separate obstetric anaesthetic team).

The Royal Colleges of Anaesthetists and The Pain Society have suggested that Acute Pain Services should have clearly defined objectives (Table 4.5). Increasingly, Acute Pain Services are dealing with ever more complex patients and the boundary between acute and non-acute (chronic) pain management has become blurred as Acute Pain Services deal with acute-on-chronic pain and persistent post-operative pain.

The delivery of an effective Acute Pain Service necessitates a robust system for patient selection, preparation (including supplying patients with information), and follow up. Daily patient ward rounds allow for adjustments to be made according to analgesic requirements and for plans to be formulated for continuation or discontinuation of analgesic techniques. Acute Pain Services should also have systems for dealing with urgent referrals and out of hours calls. In addition, analgesia should be safe and effective. This requires regular assessment and monitoring not just for respiratory depression and hypotension but also for motor block (epidural analgesia), emesis, pruritus, and nightmares/hallucinations.

Optimal acute pain management is facilitated by the provision of organizational structures for the delivery of pain relief, including guidelines (systematically developed statements to assist decisions about appropriate care for specific clinical circumstances). A number of professional organizations have produced practice guidelines for pain management. The American Society of Anesthesiologists guidelines for the management of acute post-operative pain recommend

## Table 4.5 Objectives of an Acute Pain Service

- Establishment of a system for regular assessment and treatment of acute pain
- Provision of specialist care and advice for difficult acute pain problems
- Seamless liaison with other health care teams with shared responsibility
- Provision of backup arrangements to ensure continuous cover for acute pain management
- Patient information and education
- Continuing education of all health care staff
- Continuing audit and evaluation of the service

a multimodal approach to perioperative pain management by using three specific techniques (PCA, epidural analgesia, and regional analgesia) and recognition of specific features of perioperative pain management for paediatric and geriatric patients and in ambulatory surgery. Whilst the US Public Health Service Agency for Health Care Policy and Research guidelines include a useful flow chart for the treatment of acute pain (Figure 4.1). At present, although there is anecdotal evidence in support of a beneficial effect of practice guidelines for acute pain management there are no randomized, controlled studies.

### 4.3.2 Effectiveness of Acute Pain Services

Effective treatment of acute pain is one of the most important functions of an Acute Pain Service but it is necessary to differentiate between the benefits of the analgesic techniques *per se* and the benefits

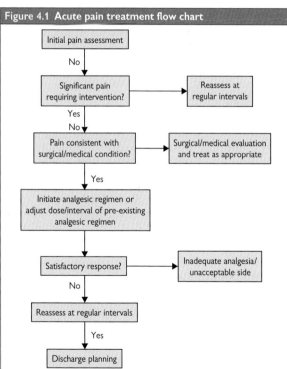

### Figure 4.1 Acute pain treatment flow chart

Initial pain assessment

↓ No

Significant pain requiring intervention? → Reassess at regular intervals

↓ Yes
↓ No

Pain consistent with surgical/medical condition? → Surgical/medical evaluation and treat as appropriate

↓ Yes

Initiate analgesic regimen or adjust dose/interval of pre-existing analgesic regimen

↓

Satisfactory response? → Inadequate analgesia/ unacceptable side

↓ No

Reassess at regular intervals

↓ Yes

Discharge planning

Adapted from Carr DB, Jacox AK, Chapman CR, et al. (1992). *Acute Pain Management: Operative or Medical Procedures and Trauma. Clinical Practice Guideline No.1. Publication 92–032.* US Public Health Service, Agency for Health Care Policy and Research, Rockville, MD. http://www.ncbi.nlm.nih.gov/books/bv.fcgi?rid=hstat6.chapter.8991 (last accessed February 2010).

35

accruing from the greater specialist supervision and education provided by the Acute Pain Services itself. There are a number of publications suggesting that anaesthesia-based Acute Pain Services are associated with an improved quality of post-operative pain management. A review of publications (predominantly audits) by Werner *et al.* (2002) suggested that Acute Pain Services were associated with improved quality of post-operative pain management, lower incidence of side effects, higher satisfaction scores, and earlier discharge from hospital. However, a subsequent systematic review of acute pain teams and the management of post-operative pain identified only 15 studies of varying quality, 9 of which included measures of pain, and only 4 of these provided suitable data for analysis. The authors concluded that there was insufficient robust research to assess the impact of Acute Pain teams on post-operative outcome or on the process of post-operative pain relief. Cost–benefit studies have been similarly difficult to perform due to the lack of well-defined baseline and outcome measures. Overall, Acute Pain Services are probably cost-effective but there is no evidence that a specialist nurse-based service is more cost-effective than an anaesthetist-led multidisciplinary team.

# References

Australian and New Zealand College of Anaesthetists and Faculty of Pain Medicine. (2005). *Acute Pain Management: Scientific Evidence*, 2nd edn. ANZCA, Melbourne. Available at http://www.anzca.edu.au/resources/books-and-publications/ (last accessed February 2010)

McDonnell A, Nicholl J, and Read SM (2003). Acute pain teams and the management of postoperative pain: a systematic review and meta-analysis. *Journal of Advanced Nursing*, **41**, 261–73.

Royal Colleges of Surgeons of England and College of Anaesthetists. Commission on the provision of surgical services. (1990). *Report of the Working Party of Pain after Surgery*. Royal Colleges of Surgeons, London.

Royal College of Anaesthetists and Pain Society. (2003). *Pain Management Services. Good Practice*. Royal College of Anaesthetists, London.

Werner MU, Søholm L, Rotbøll-Nielson P, and Kehlet H (2002). Does an acute pain service improve postoperative outcome? *Anesthesia & Analgesia*, **95**, 1361–72.

# Chapter 5

# Evidence and outcomes in acute pain management

Suellen M. Walker

> ## Key points
>
> - Inadequate control of post-operative pain can be associated with acute morbidity and have adverse effects on recovery and emotional well-being.
> - The aims of acute pain medicine are reducing pain intensity, control of side effects, hastening rehabilitation, and improving acute and long-term outcomes.
> - League tables compare the efficacy of analgesics, based on the number-needed-to-treat (NNT) to achieve 50% pain reduction.
> - Systematic reviews of different interventions for acute pain are conducted and regularly updated in the Cochrane Library.
> - The second edition of *Acute Pain Management: Scientific Evidence* by the Australian and New Zealand College of Anaesthetists and Faculty of Pain Medicine provides a useful summary of the current evidence.

## 5.1 Introduction

With advances in medical care and the introduction of new therapies, the number of clinical trials investigating treatments for acute pain has increased exponentially. As a result, there has been increasing reliance on systematic reviews and meta-analyses to synthesize current evidence, and a great deal of information is now accessible and widely available on the Internet. League tables compare the efficacy of analgesics, based on the number-needed-to-treat (NNT) to achieve 50% pain reduction (www.jr2.ox.ac.uk/bandolier/booth/painpag/Acutrev/Analgesics/Leagtab.html). Systematic reviews of different interventions for acute pain are conducted and regularly updated in the Cochrane Library (www3.interscience.wiley.com/cgi-bin/mrwhome/106568753/HOME). Current evidence for acute pain management, including but not limited to post-operative pain, and in specific patient groups, is summarized in the second edition of *Acute Pain Management: Scientific Evidence* by the Australian and New Zealand College of Anaesthetists and Faculty of Pain Medicine (www.anzca.edu.au/publications/acutepain.htm). More detailed procedure-specific recommendations for the perioperative period are being developed by the PROSPECT group (www.postoppain.org). These encompass not only analgesic efficacy data, but also information relating to anaesthetic and surgical management, and emphasize a multimodal rehabilitative approach. However, the aim of evidence-based guidelines is not to provide global standards or absolute requirements, but to assist decision-making about health care. The use of guidelines cannot guarantee any specific outcome, and clinicians must evaluate the evidence within the context of their expertise and their practice setting, with consideration of the risks, benefits, and treatment preferences of individual patients.

This chapter briefly summarizes data obtained from recent systematic reviews and meta-analyses investigating the effect of perioperative analgesia on pain, morbidity, and general health outcomes in adults. Obstetric and paediatric patients are the subjects of other chapters.

## 5.2 **Pain-related outcomes**

### 5.2.1 Intensity

A reduction in pain intensity is often the primary outcome in analgesic trials. This may be measured on categorical verbal descriptor scales (e.g. none, mild, moderate, severe) or with a numerical rating scale (e.g. 0–10 visual analogue scale [VAS]). Statistically significant changes are reported in clinical trials, but may not always correlate with a clinically significant change for individual patients. A reduction in pain intensity by 30–35% has been rated as clinically meaningful by adult patients with post-operative pain or acute pain in the emergency department. Meta-analyses of pain intensity or pain relief measures can be used to derive the NNT for one patient to achieve a given outcome (e.g. at least 50% pain relief), thus allowing evaluation and comparison of the efficacy of different agents.

#### 5.2.1.1 *PCA versus conventional analgesia*

Patient-controlled analgesia (PCA) most often refers to the intravenous administration of opioids, although efficacy has also been shown for other routes (e.g. subcutaneous or regional), and new preparations (e.g. transdermal and inhaled) are becoming available. PCA provides better pain control and greater patient satisfaction than parenteral 'as-needed' (i.e. conventional) administration of opioids.

Although statistically significant, the clinical significance of the improvement in pain scores (i.e. 8-point lowering in 1–100 VAS score) has been questioned. However, the success of conventional analgesia is dependent on staff availability and avoiding delays in administration, and PCA may have additional advantages in terms of staff time and patient preference. With appropriate dosing and programming, no major differences have been found in the efficacy of different opioids via PCA, but individual patients may tolerate one opioid more than another.

### 5.2.1.2 *Epidural versus parenteral analgesia*
Direct comparisons between parenteral PCA and epidural analgesia are difficult. Analysis of controlled trials may be biased by inadequate blinding; incomplete recording of all side effects or outcomes; heterogeneous patient groups undergoing different types of surgery; publication of only positive studies; and inclusion of older smaller trials which overestimate the therapeutic effect in meta-analyses. Epidural analgesia improves analgesia (at rest and with movement) for up to 3 days after intra-abdominal surgery. After abdominal aortic aneurysm (AAA) surgery, analgesia is improved (most markedly for pain on movement), regardless of the level of insertion or type of epidural drug used. Early analgesia is also improved by epidural analgesia after lower limb joint replacement, but no difference from PCA was detectable by 18–24hr.

### 5.2.2 **Analgesic consumption**
A reduction in analgesic consumption may be used as a measure of analgesic efficacy, when comparing two routes of administration or when an active versus placebo drug is added to an analgesic regime. The clinical significance of any change will depend on demonstration of either improved efficacy with the combination or a reduction in side effects as lower doses of each drug are effective in combination, without the introduction of new side effects.

When comparing PCA and conventional analgesia, improvements in efficacy are associated with higher opioid consumption. However, the increase is relatively small (six morphine equivalents in first 24hr; about 30% more) and is associated with an increase in itch, but no change in post-operative nausea and vomiting (PONV). The incidence of respiratory depression has not been found to differ between PCA and conventional analgesia, although methods of evaluating and reporting differences vary across studies. There is little evidence for benefit of epidural opioid alone over systemic opioid administration for acute pain. However, combination of epidural opioid and local anaesthetic improves analgesia, and reduces local anaesthetic requirements and side effects when compared with local anaesthetic alone.

Ketamine decreases both opioid consumption and pain score, and an associated reduction in PONV has been shown in some studies. Psychomimetic side effects of ketamine may be apparent after administration in awake or sedated patients with regional anaesthesia, but are rare when administered in conjunction with general anaesthesia. Non-steroidal anti-inflammatory drugs (NSAIDs) decrease opioid requirements by 30–40% and there is increasing evidence of an associated decrease in opioid-related PONV and sedation. This may occur at the cost of an increased risk of bleeding which can be important after some surgical procedures. The risk of bleeding is related to altered platelet function, which in itself varies from drug to drug. Aspirin caused irreversible changes in platelets, whereas some non-steroidals such as dexketoprofen are said to produce minimal effects on bleeding. Reductions in opioid consumption are less marked with the addition of paracetamol (approximately 20%), and reductions in side effects have not been confirmed.

### 5.2.3 Global satisfaction

When compared with conventional analgesia, PCA has been associated with improvements in both the degree of satisfaction in individual patients and in the proportion of patients satisfied. This was apparent even in early studies that failed to show an improvement in pain score, suggesting that factors such as patient control and reduced fear of inadequate analgesia may be contributing factors. Global satisfaction scores may also be influenced by the incidence and severity of side effects, a desire to please health care staff, the mood and coping style of individual patients, and the level of communication. As a result, satisfaction alone is not a suitable measure for assessing the efficacy of analgesia.

### 5.2.4 Duration of analgesia or pain

An analgesic intervention has a 'preventive effect' if it produces an impact on pain score and/or analgesic consumption that extends beyond the expected clinical duration of action of the drug. Positive preventive effects have been demonstrated for NMDA antagonists (ketamine and dextromethorphan), local anaesthetic techniques (epidural and peripheral nerve block), and NSAIDs, but not opioids. Preventive effects have also been reported with gabapentin, although the required dose and duration of treatment require clarification. In contrast, there is mixed but not conclusive evidence of positive 'pre-emptive' analgesic effects, which relate solely to the timing of the analgesic intervention (i.e. preincisional versus post-incisional administration improves efficacy).

The presence of *pre*operative pain and the intensity of early *post*-operative pain have been identified as risk factors for persistent pain after surgery. Improved management of early analgesia has been associated with a lower incidence of persistent pain in some high-risk surgeries (e.g. after thoracotomy and mastectomy), but there is conflicting data about the impact of perioperative analgesia on post-amputation pain.

## 5.3 Morbidity and mortality

As clinical practice changes with time, it can be difficult to accurately assess the impact of analgesic interventions on morbidity and mortality. Improvements in perioperative care and monitoring, the use of short-acting anaesthetic agents, and improved thromboprophylaxis have all had an impact on respiratory, cardiovascular, and thromboembolic complications. In addition, there have been alterations in surgical management, with less invasive procedures, and adoption of a rehabilitative approach with earlier ambulation and enteral nutrition. Whereas early trials reported a range of benefits with epidural analgesia, more recent studies have failed to show major impacts on morbidity or mortality. Combining data in meta-analyses does not provide all the answers as the prevalence of relatively rare complications (e.g. post-operative death) may not be accurately reflected and the reporting of side effects can vary across individual studies. No difference in mortality could be demonstrated with epidural versus parenteral analgesia in a large trial of high-risk patients, or in recent meta-analyses of trials after major abdominal surgery. Restricting the analysis to trials with similar surgical procedures may make differences in morbidity more apparent (e.g. epidural analgesia reduces cardiac complications after AAA surgery), but if patient numbers are too low, potential differences in complication rates may not be apparent (e.g. after lower limb surgery). The relative effects of analgesia on interrelated outcomes may also be difficult to evaluate. For example, a decrease in pain on coughing will have an impact on respiratory complications, whereas earlier extubation may be associated with earlier ambulation and enteral nutrition.

Clinical practice requires consideration of the individual as well as the evidence obtained from population studies. Evaluation of the relative risks, as well as the benefits, of different analgesic regimes is required. Neurological complications are rare after epidural analgesia but may have devastating effects for the individual. As a result, the PROSPECT group recommend parenteral analgesia rather than epidural analgesia for low-risk patients undergoing abdominal hysterectomy. The relative importance of side effects may differ for individual patients. For example, PCA has been associated with a higher incidence of pruritus, but was this associated with a significant degree of discomfort? Individuals may reduce their PCA demands to minimize opioid-related side effects (particularly PONV), even at the expense of increased pain.

### 5.3.1 **Morbidity and complications**

#### 5.3.1.1 *Gastrointestinal side effects*

Variable reporting of side effects such as PONV make it difficult to adequately compare effects of different analgesics in a meta-analysis. After intra-abdominal surgery or lower limb joint replacement, the incidence of PONV did not differ in patients receiving epidural or parenteral opioid analgesia. The clinical impact of PONV may be more accurately reflected by its severity (frequency and duration) than the overall incidence.

In early analyses, epidural analgesia was associated with improvements in bowel motility (without any increase in dehiscence) and an earlier return of gastrointestinal function. This has not been confirmed in later studies, but these results may also be influenced by changes in surgical management.

#### 5.3.1.2 *Respiratory complications*

The incidence of respiratory depression is difficult to determine as definitions and monitoring techniques vary in different centres and across clinical trials. No difference in the incidence of respiratory depression has been identified in meta-analyses comparing PCA and conventional analgesia, or PCA and epidural analgesia. Early analysis showed a reduction in pulmonary complications with epidural analgesia (local anaesthetic greater than opioid) compared with parenteral opioid. Respiratory failure was less common after epidural versus PCA in high-risk patients undergoing major abdominal surgery; but no difference could be demonstrated after lower limb joint replacement. The duration of tracheal intubation and mechanical ventilation was reduced by thoracic, but not lumbar epidural analgesia after AAA repair, but there was no difference in the incidence of pneumonia.

#### 5.3.1.3 *Cardiovascular complications*

The incidence of myocardial infarction was lower with thoracic, but not lumbar, epidural analgesia when compared with systemic opioid after AAA repair. Overall, early reports of improved cardiac morbidity with epidural analgesia have not been confirmed in subsequent large controlled trials.

Improved thromboprophylaxis has decreased the clinical impact of analgesic regimes on the frequency of deep venous thrombosis.

## 5.4 **General health and functional outcomes**

A multidisciplinary rehabilitative approach has been proposed to improve post-operative outcome. This aims to maximize dynamic pain relief (i.e. pain on movement and coughing) and modify surgical practice to ensure early ambulation, enteral feeding, and hasten return to normal function. The PROSPECT group emphasize the need to base treatment choices on the type of surgery being performed, as pain and organ dysfunction vary with different procedures. For example, pain on coughing after thoracotomy may have a major influence on respiratory outcomes, and ileus after abdominal surgery will produce specific effects on catabolism and nutrition.

Although functional outcomes are important for the assessment of the patient's overall recovery, they are often not reported and there is no standardized use of measurement tools. In 13 studies after lower limb joint replacement, only 3 assessed functional outcome, but all used a different measure and the clinical significance of the reported changes was not clear.

Length of hospital stay is an important outcome not only for patients, but also for health care agencies when the cost of different treatments is being evaluated. No difference in hospital stay has been confirmed with PCA versus conventional opioid or with epidural versus PCA. However, administrative and social factors can have a greater impact on discharge criteria than the quality of post-operative analgesia.

Patient-based assessment of recovery and convalescence is important for the evaluation of overall health care. Multiple factors will influence the quality and speed of recovery including physical and cognitive functioning; mental health; symptoms such as pain and PONV; sleep disturbance; and energy levels. A large number of tools are available for assessing health-related quality of life, but many have been developed for specific disease processes (e.g. rheumatoid arthritis), and are more often used to evaluate patients with chronic rather than acute pain conditions. A recent systematic review recommended the 40-item Quality of Recovery score questionnaire (QoR-40) as the most robust tool currently available. Standardized use of this measure would facilitate comparison across clinical trials.

Psychological factors, such as preoperative preparation and education, expectations, mood (i.e. anxiety or depression), and coping style (e.g. catastrophizing), can influence the patient's report of pain and analgesic consumption (e.g. number of PCA demands). Although studies vary in their quality and methodology, positive correlations have been reported between preoperative anxiety and catastrophizing and subsequent pain. In addition, unrelieved pain will influence psychological well-being and may have an impact on the recovery and the response to future interventions. These factors require further evaluation in clinical acute pain trials.

# References

Block BM, Liu SS, Rowlingson AJ, Cowan AR, Cowan JA Jr, and Wu CL (2003). Efficacy of postoperative epidural analgesia: a meta-analysis. *JAMA*, **290**, 2455–63.

Choi PT, Bhandari M, Scott J, and Douketis J (2003). Epidural analgesia for pain relief following hip or knee replacement. *Cochrane Database of Systematic Reviews*, **2003**, CD003071.

Elia N and Tramer MR (2005). Ketamine and postoperative pain—a quantitative systematic review of randomised trials. *Pain*, **113**, 61–70.

Elia N, Lysakowski C, and Tramer MR (2005). Does multimodal analgesia with acetaminophen, nonsteroidal antiinflammatory drugs, or selective cyclooxygenase-2 inhibitors and patient-controlled analgesia morphine offer advantages over morphine alone? Meta-analyses of randomized trials. *Anesthesiology*, **103**, 1296–304.

Granot M and Ferber SG (2005). The roles of pain catastrophizing and anxiety in the prediction of postoperative pain intensity: a prospective study. *Clinical Journal of Pain*, **21**, 439–45.

Herrera FJ, Wong J, and Chung F (2007). A systematic review of postoperative recovery outcomes measurements after ambulatory surgery. *Anesthesia & Analgesics*, **105**, 63–9.

Hudcova J, McNicol E, Quah C, *et al.* (2006). Patient controlled opioid analgesia versus conventional opioid analgesia for postoperative pain. *Cochrane Database of Systematic Reviews*, **2006**, CD003348.

Mauermann WJ, Shilling AM, and Zuo Z (2006). A comparison of neuraxial block versus general anesthesia for elective total hip replacement: a meta-analysis. *Anesthesia & Analgesics*, **103**, 1018–25.

McCartney CJ, Sinha A, and Katz J (2004). A qualitative systematic review of the role of N-methyl-D-aspartate receptor antagonists in preventive analgesia. *Anesthesia & Analgesics*, **98**, 1385–400.

Nishimori M, Ballantyne JC, and Low JH (2006). Epidural pain relief versus systemic opioid-based pain relief for abdominal aortic surgery. *Cochrane Database of Systematic Reviews*, **2006**, CD005059.

Ong CK, Lirk P, Seymour RA, and Jenkins BJ (2005). The efficacy of preemptive analgesia for acute postoperative pain management: a meta-analysis. *Anesthesia & Analgesics*, **100**, 757–73.

Werawatganon T and Charuluxanun S (2005). Patient controlled intravenous opioid analgesia versus continuous epidural analgesia for pain after intra-abdominal surgery. *Cochrane Database of Systematic Reviews*, **2005**, CD004088.

Wu CL, Cohen SR, Richman JM, *et al.* (2005). Efficacy of postoperative patient-controlled and continuous infusion epidural analgesia versus intravenous patient-controlled analgesia with opioids: a meta-analysis. *Anesthesiology*, **103**, 1079–88.

## Chapter 6

# Post-operative pain

Elizabeth Ashley and Mano Doraiswami

> **Key points**
>
> - Pain relief is a basic human right.
> - Pain has detrimental acute and chronic effects on the physiology and psychology of patients.
> - Inadequately controlled pain can cause post-operative morbidity, prolong recovery time, increase the use of health care resources, thereby increasing total health care costs.
> - Post-operative pain is most effectively managed with a multimodal approach.

## 6.1 The principles of post-operative pain management

The management of post-operative pain was not considered to be a priority until relatively recently. In the developed world, it is now acknowledged that treating post-operative pain has a positive effect on the time taken to recover from surgery, but in large parts of the world little or no provision is made in terms of drugs or personnel to relive suffering after surgery and to thereby enhance recovery.

Initially, the interest in post-operative pain began in the United States and in the United Kingdom. The Joint Report of the Royal Colleges of Surgeons and Anaesthetists, published in 1990, highlighted the need to manage post-operative pain more effectively.

Early audits showed that up to 80% of patients were in severe pain in the first 48hr post-operatively. Introduction of simple measures such as routinely measuring pain scores, and using algorithms for frequent use of intramuscular morphine were effective in reducing incidence of severe pain. The report recommended the introduction of multidisciplinary pain teams, and this has now become the norm in most UK acute hospitals. The subsequent introduction of patient-controlled analgesia (PCA) devices, and routine use of epidurals for post-operative pain have been achieved largely through acute pain teams. The original concept intended the team to consist of surgeons, anaesthetists, and nurses, 18yrs on from the report, the presence of surgeons on the team is the exception rather than the rule, but there is great surgical interest in the use of enhance recovery plans, in which pain management plays a vital part.

## 6.1.1 Physiological effects of pain

The rationale for treating post-operative pain is based on three pre-cepts: first, to relieve suffering of the patient; second, to avoid the adverse physiological effects caused by pain; and third, to avoid the adverse psychological effects. In addition, there is increasing evidence that reducing acute post-operative pain reduces the incidence of chronic pain. The adverse physiological effects can be seen in many different systems.

### 6.1.1.1 *Cardiovascular system*

Pain activates the sympathetic nervous system causing an increase in heart rate and blood pressure, resulting in an increase in myocardial oxygen consumption and decreased time for oxygen delivery. This is especially harmful in patients with pre-existing ischaemic heart disease.

### 6.1.1.2 *Respiratory system*

Pain decreases the ability to deep breathe and cough effectively (especially after upper abdominal and thoracic operations), causing decreased lung volume and functional residual capacity leading to basal atelectasis, sputum retention, and increased risk of respiratory infection.

### 6.1.1.3 *Gastrointestinal system*

An increase in sympathetic activity caused by pain results in a reduc-tion in smooth muscle tone of the gastrointestinal tract and diversion of blood flow to vital organs leading to decreased gut motility and to post-operative ileus. Untreated acute pain can cause nausea and vomiting.

### 6.1.1.4 *Thromboembolic*

Decreased movement and immobilization due to pain may increase the risk of thromboembolic events.

### 6.1.1.5 *Stress response*

The neurohormonal response to pain involves the hypothalamic, pituitary, adrenocortical, and sympathoadrenal interactions.

Pain increases sympathetic activity leading to catecholamine secre-tion from the adrenals and catabolic hormone secretion from the pituitary gland. The effects are increased metabolism and catabolism leading to increased oxygen consumption, increase in blood glucose, free fatty acids, ketone bodies, and lactate. The secretion of antidiu-retic hormone results in sodium and water retention. Attenuation of the stress response caused by post-operative pain may facilitate and accelerate the patient's recovery post-operatively.

### 6.1.2 Psychological effects of pain

Acute post-operative pain may result in anxiety, fear, sleep disturbances, depression, and a feeling of helplessness. The fear and anxiety can lead to 'avoidance behaviour' leading to decreased physical activity. Anxiety can augment the sympathetic activity evoked by acute pain. The level of preoperative anxiety is correlated to the perception of post-operative pain.

### 6.1.3 Acute to chronic pain

Neuropathic pain is defined as pain initiated or caused by a primary dysfunction in the peripheral or central nervous system.

Although a cause of chronic pain, neuropathic pain is now recognized as a cause of acute post-surgical pain. There is a high risk of acute neuropathic pain progressing to chronic pain.

Chronic pain is relatively common after procedures such as limb amputation, thoracotomy, sternotomy, breast surgery, hernia repair, and gallbladder surgery. Studies suggest that the severity of acute post-operative pain may be an important predictor in the development of chronic pain. Continued peripheral nociceptive stimulus from surgical injury causes central sensitization and chronic pain. The prevention of central sensitization and control of post-operative pain may decrease the incidence of chronic pain (Table 6.1).

| Table 6.1 Risk factors for the development of chronic post-surgical pain |
| --- |
| **Preoperative factors** |
| • Pain, moderate to severe, lasting more than a month |
| • Repeat surgery |
| • Psychological vulnerability |
| **Intraoperative factors** |
| • Surgery involving nerve damage, surgical site, for example, thoracic surgery and breast surgery |
| **Post-operative factors** |
| • Moderate to severe pain |
| • Depression |
| • Anxiety |
| • Neuroticism |

## 6.2 Management of post-operative pain

### 6.2.1 Introduction

The management of post-operative pain starts before the surgery is performed. The preoperative consultation by the anaesthetist will include a discussion of the plan for managing post-operative pain. Histories of any previous operations, the way pain has been managed in the past, and the quality of previous pain relief are established. The patient is provided with information about the options for pain relief, and if an epidural is being considered then an informed consent must be obtained. Any contraindications or previous adverse reactions to analgesic drugs are established. If drugs are to be administered *per rectum* information is given and consent obtained.

In the post-operative period, a multidisciplinary team should run the acute pain service with responsibilities for managing post-operative pain, training medical and nursing staff, research, and audit.

The basis of pain management has three elements:

- Assessment of pain
- Treatment of pain
- Reassessment of pain and pain relief.

The commonest reason for undertreatment of pain is the failure to assess pain and pain relief. Assessment of pain should be done at frequent and regular intervals and should be documented. Pain measurement should be recorded on the TPR (temperature, pulse, and respiration) chart as part of the routine observations of all patients.

Treatment of pain should be based on local protocols and guidelines (e.g. analgesic ladder, PCA, epidural protocols, etc.). Written protocols will guide the medical and nursing personnel to institute appropriate management (see example in Figure 6.1).

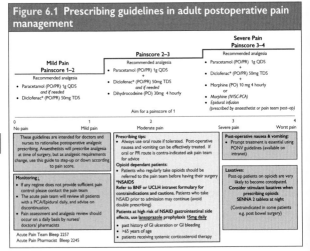

### Figure 6.1 Prescribing guidelines in adult postoperative pain management

**Mild Pain** — Painscore 1–2
Recommended analgesia
- Paracetamol (PO/PR) 1g QDS *and if needed*
- Diclofenac* (PO/PR) 50mg TDS

**Painscore 2–3**
Recommended analgesia
- Paracetamol (PO/PR) 1g QDS
- Diclofenac* (PO/PR) 50mg TDS *and if needed*
- Dihydrocodeine (PO) 30mg 4 hourly

**Severe Pain** — Painscore 3–4
Recommended analgesia
- Paracetamol (PO/PR) 1g QDS
- Diclofenac* (PO/PR) 50mg TDS
- Morphine (PO) 10 mg 4 hourly *or*
- Morphine (IV/SC-PCA)
- Epidural infusion
(prescribed by anaesthetist or pain team post-op)

Aim for a painscore of 1

| 0 | 1 | 2 | 3 | 4 |
|---|---|---|---|---|
| No pain | Mild pain | Moderate pain | Severe pain | Worst pain |

These guidelines are intended for doctors and nurses to rationalise postoperative analgesic prescribing. Anaesthetists will prescribe analgesia at time of surgery, but as analgesic requirements change, use this guide to step-up or down according to pain score.

**Prescribing tips:**
- Always use oral route if tolerated. Post-operative nausea and vomiting can be effectively treated. If oral or PR route is contra-indicated ask pain team for advice

**Opioid dependant patients:**
- Patients who regularly take opioids should be referred to the pain team before having their surgery

**Post-operative nausea & vomiting:**
- Prompt treatment is essential using PONV guidelines (available on intranet)

**Monitoring:**
- If any regime does not provide sufficient pain control please contact the pain team
- The acute pain team will review all patients with a PCA/Epidural daily, and advise on discontinuation.
- Pain assessment and analgesia review should occur on a daily basis by nurses/ doctors/ pharmacists

Acute Pain Team Bleep 2257
Acute Pain Pharmacist Bleep 2245

**\*NSAIDS**
Refer to BNF or UCLH intranet formulary for contraindications and cautions. Patients who take NSAID prior to admission may continue (avoid double prescribing)
Patients at high risk of NSAID gastrointestinal side effects, use lansoprazole prophylaxis 15mg daily
- past history of GI ulceration or GI bleeding
- >65 years of age
- patients receiving systemic corticosteroid therapy

**Laxatives:**
Post-op patients on opioids are very likely to become constipated.
**Consider stimulant laxatives when prescribing opioids**
SENNA 2 tablets at night
(Contraindicated in some patients e.g. post bowel surgery)

The acute pain team is not intended to take over the management of pain in all the post-operative patients. Surgical and nursing staff should be trained to a level of competence that allows them to manage routine post-operative pain. However, the pain team will visit any patient referred to them by ward staff where pain control is difficult and give advice. The acute pain team should assess everyday all patients on intravenous PCA or epidural infusion. Designated personnel should be available 24hr a day commonly, this is arranged so that acute pain nurses are available in the day and anaesthetic trainees at night.

### 6.2.2 Measurement of post-operative pain

Pain is a subjective experience and there is no satisfactory objective measurement of pain. Pain measurement tools can be unidimensional or multidimensional. In most post-operative pain services, unidimentional scales have been adopted. Numerical rating scales are used for adults where the patient rates the pain from 0 to 10, 0 being no pain and 10 being worst possible pain. A scale of 0–4 can also be used. It Is valuable to have a consistent use of either 0–10 or 0–4 across the whole hospital to reduce confusion and to aid the audit of the service.

A visual analogue scale (VAS), where the patient marks the severity of pain on a 100mm line, is more commonly used as a research tool as it is cumbersome to use as a routine.

For young children, mentally impaired and patients with communication difficulties, a picture (faces) scale is commonly used. The picture scale consists of a series of faces from a happy, smiling face to a sad and crying face.

### 6.2.3 Options for post-operative pain management

The goal for post-operative pain management is to reduce or eliminate pain and discomfort with minimal side effects.

Treatment available for acute post-operative pain ranges from simple analgesics to more complex interventions such as central neuraxial blockade (epidural infusions), PCA techniques, and peripheral nerve blockade.

Post-operative pain occurs by different mechanisms (nociceptive, inflammatory, and neuropathic). Monotherapy will act on one of the pathways of pain whereas multimodal analgesia acts on multiple pain pathways.

Multimodal analgesia uses different analgesics and techniques in combination to get maximum pain relief whilst reducing the adverse effects of the individual drugs and techniques. Multimodal analgesia, which allows early mobilization of patients, can reduce hospital stay.

The principle characteristic of post-operative pain is that it is at its most intense immediately after the surgery and the intensity diminishes over the subsequent days and weeks. Therefore in managing post-operative pain, we could consider that the analgesic ladder is stepped down rather than up. We start with the potent opioids and expect to step down to intermediate strength drugs and finally the patient will be comfortable with simple analgesics. The purpose of the multimodal approach is to use all three classes of analgesics at the beginning when pain is most intense in order to minimize the dosage of each drug and therefore reduce side effects. As the pain lessens, the most potent class of drug is removed, and replaced by less potent drugs until the patient is pain free.

The opioid drug given in the post-operative period is commonly morphine or fentanyl. The most common methods of delivery are by the epidural route in combination with local anaesthetic, by intravenous injection as a continuous infusion in a high dependence area, or by an intravenous PCA device.

Where non-steroidal anti-inflammatory drugs can be tolerated they can be given intravenously during surgery, *per rectum* whilst the patient is nil by mouth, and then orally.

Paracetamol is given throughout the post-operative period when not contraindicated. It can be given intravenously, rectally, or orally as appropriate.

### 6.2.4 **Patient-controlled analgesia**

The principle of PCA is that the patient should administer analgesia when they feel the pain is sufficient to justify further drug. This broad principle does not define the route by which the drug is given, but in common use the phrase PCA has come to refer to either intravenous or epidural (PCEA) administration. In standard intravenous PCA, the most commonly used drug is morphine, a 1mg bolus, with a 5min lockout time. The alternative is fentanyl 20mcg with a 5min lockout time. This is commonly prescribed using a preprinted sticker that can be fixed to the drug chart. Supplementary oxygen, usually by Hudson mask or nasal cannula, should also be prescribed and administered while opiates are being delivered. Naloxone may also be prescribed for use if the respiratory rate falls below a given rate, frequently five breaths per minute.

A dedicated intravenous access is required for intravenous PCA, anti-siphon valves are used to prevent siphoning of the drug into the patient by the intravenous infusion back flow into the line. Antireflux or one-way valves ensure that the drug goes into the patient.

Monitoring of the patient and recording of observations are key safety features. Regular pain scores, respiratory rate, and sedation score should be recorded. The pain team will record the total consumption of drug and the dose/demand ratio, these are available from the pump. These may guide adjustments to the regime.

Anti-emetics should be prescribed with intravenous PCA, this can also be done using a preprinted sticker. The most common side effect of intravenous PCA is nausea and vomiting, which may be severe enough to prevent adequate analgesia. More than one anti-emetic should be prescribed, choosing drugs with different mechanisms of action. This allows nursing staff to adjust the anti-emetic according to response.

### 6.2.5 Epidural analgesia

Epidural analgesia is the gold standard for post-operative pain, providing better analgesia than parenteral opioid administration, both in terms of pain relief and side effect profile. Placing an epidural is invasive and carries some serious risks associated with placing a catheter into the epidural space. The risk benefit is positive in the case of major abdominal and thoracic surgeries, and may be justified for major lower limb surgery. An epidural would not be justified for abdominal surface surgery unless the patient co-morbidities altered the risk benefit ratio, for example, in a patient with severe respiratory disease, because epidural analgesia improves oxygenation and reduces pulmonary complications compared with parenteral opioids. Epidural infusions also decrease the incidence of venous thromboembolism, especially after orthopaedic surgery due to vasodilatation.

Epidural analgesia can be given by continuous infusion or by epidural PCA. The infusion given may be an opioid alone, local anaesthetic alone, or a combination of the two drugs. Opiates alone do not provide good quality analgesia. A combination of local anaesthetic and opioids in the epidural space are synergistic, providing the best quality of analgesia. On occasions where pain is difficult to manage, local anaesthetic alone may be given, and opiates given by a different route. A commonly used mixture is bupivacaine or levobupivacaine 0.1–0.125% and 2mcg/mL of fentanyl. Diamorphine and preservative-free morphine are also used.

Monitoring of patients with epidural infusion should include pulse, blood pressure, respiratory rate, $SaO_2$, level of block, sedation score, pain score, and any untoward adverse events. The epidural site should be inspected for leaks, catheter dislodgement, and signs of infection (i.e. redness, fluctuance, and pain on palpation).

Adverse effects of epidural analgesia include high block, profound motor block, hypotension, respiratory depression, nausea and vomiting, pruritus, and urinary retention.

If a high block occurs, the infusion should be stopped or the infusion rate decreased, vital signs should be closely monitored, hypotension should be treated with intravenous fluids, vasopressors (ephedrine or metraminol boluses), and block regression monitored.

If respiratory depression occurs, block level should be checked, infusion should be stopped, and naloxone given. Oxygen should be supplemented throughout the duration of the epidural infusion.

Epidural analgesia fails because of catheter displacement, inadequate dose, and leakage. Epidural rescue protocols are helpful in the management of failed epidurals (see Figure 6.2).

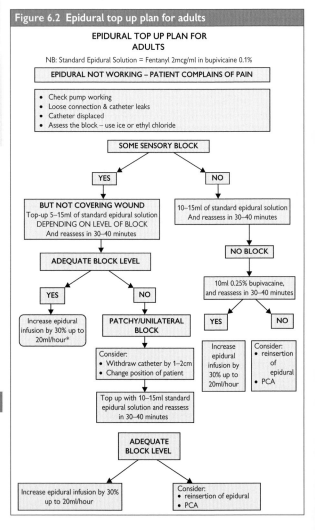

**Figure 6.2 Epidural top up plan for adults**

EPIDURAL TOP UP PLAN FOR ADULTS

NB: Standard Epidural Solution = Fentanyl 2mcg/ml in bupivicaine 0.1%

EPIDURAL NOT WORKING – PATIENT COMPLAINS OF PAIN

- Check pump working
- Loose connection & catheter leaks
- Catheter displaced
- Assess the block – use ice or ethyl chloride

SOME SENSORY BLOCK

YES → BUT NOT COVERING WOUND
Top-up 5–15ml of standard epidural solution DEPENDING ON LEVEL OF BLOCK And reassess in 30–40 minutes

ADEQUATE BLOCK LEVEL

YES → Increase epidural infusion by 30% up to 20ml/hour*

NO → PATCHY/UNILATERAL BLOCK
Consider:
- Withdraw catheter by 1–2cm
- Change position of patient

Top up with 10–15ml standard epidural solution and reassess in 30–40 minutes

NO → 10–15ml of standard epidural solution And reassess in 30–40 minutes

NO BLOCK

10ml 0.25% bupivicaine, and reassess in 30–40 minutes

YES → Increase epidural infusion by 30% up to 20ml/hour

NO → Consider:
- reinsertion of epidural
- PCA

ADEQUATE BLOCK LEVEL

Increase epidural infusion by 30% up to 20ml/hour

Consider:
- reinsertion of epidural
- PCA

Epidural PCA is used in some centres. The advantage of PCEA is that it uses lower doses of the drugs when compared with continuous epidural infusions.

The pain relief and the side effects are similar to that of continuous epidural infusion.

A continuous background infusion is often added to PCEA but does not provide superior analgesia compared to bolus PCEA only.

### 6.2.6 Local anaesthetic infusions

The improvement in the technology of producing fine bore plastic catheters, combined with a desire to minimize the side effects from systemic opiates has lead to an increasing use of indwelling post-operative catheters for local anaesthetic infusion. This technique has been used in orthopaedic surgery for pain relief after shoulder surgery, where it facilitates early physiotherapy. The technique can also be used to apply local anaesthetic to the femoral nerve, the catheter being inserted under ultrasound guidance, and can be applied to other nerve sheaths. Continuous infusions of bupivacaine, levobupivacaine, or ropivacaine are used (bupivacaine 0.25% maximum of 40mL in 24hr for hip catheter infusion is a typical regime). Modern catheters with multiple small holes along their length allow the local anaesthetic solution to be infused into the length of the wound, and some success has been achieved placing the catheter in the rectus sheath when closing a laparotomy incision, and running a continuous infusion for pain relief. This technique is valuable where an epidural cannot be placed for any reason.

Some surgeons have reservations about leaving catheters in the wound, considering the risk of wound infection to be increased. There is no evidence of increased wound infection with the use of these catheters.

### 6.2.7 Complex post-operative pain

The patient who presents for elective surgery with no history of previous operations and no history of chronic pain, who is well prepared before hand, and has straightforward surgery can expect to be pain free at rest and have mild pain on movement in the days immediately post-operatively. Where a patient has had multiple previous surgeries, with a memory of previous poor pain control, or has chronic pain, or has been taking analgesics regularly for the surgical condition, post-operative management may not be so straightforward. The preoperative history is important in these cases; a record must be made of the regular analgesic consumption before surgery. Where this includes strong or weak opiates, this regular intake should be converted to morphine and added to the expected requirements in the post-operative period. This may mean using a continuous infusion as a background to PCA and may also necessitate a change in bolus size from the standard 1mg. To allay anxiety, an analgesic plan should be made with the patient before surgery with appropriate steps up planned if required.

Where an epidural would be appropriate, an infusion of plain bupivacaine via the epidural, with the opiate requirement given by a combination of background infusion and PCA, may provide the best analgesia.

Adjuvant analgesics such as ketamine or gabapentin may be of value in these patients. Subanaesthetic doses of ketamine have shown to decrease opioid requirements, decrease pain scores, and possibly prevent the development of opioid tolerance.

In patients with morphine-resistant pain, the addition of small single dose of ketamine can provide a rapid and sustained improvement of analgesia. Clonidine enhances analgesia for post-operative pain whether given by oral, intravenous, intramuscular, epidural, intrathecal, or intra-articular routes. It is associated with marked sedation in some patients.

## 6.3 Post-operative pain management in ITU

The challenge of acute pain management in the ITU lies in the difficulty of assessing pain in patients who are intubated and sedated. Where muscle relaxants are used, there is a danger that patients may be in pain but unable to respond in any way. The distinction between sedation and analgesia may become indistinct.

Many patients in the ITU setting will not be able to use intravenous PCA machines. Alternative methods are required to ensure good pain relief.

### 6.3.1 Analgesic delivery systems in ITU

#### 6.3.1.1 *Continuous intravenous opioid infusion*

This is the method of choice in most intensive care units, because it is the commonest means of drug delivery in ITU. The continuous haemodynamic and respiratory monitoring and the one to one nursing ratio in ITU makes continuous opioid infusions a safe option.

Short-acting opioid (remifentanil and fentanyl) are used in intubated patients who are expected to be extubated within a few hours. Longer-acting opioids (e.g. morphine) are used when a prolonged period of intubation is anticipated.

#### 6.3.1.2 *Continuous epidural/perineural local anaesthetics infusion*

Epidural analgesia has many advantages for the ITU patients. The continuous infusion of a mixture of local anaesthetics and opioids, as used on the wards can also be used in ITU. The advantages of reduced risk of deep vein thrombosis, and better respiratory function may be very important for patients who are in long-term intensive care, or are being weaned from mechanical ventilation.

Haemodynamic instability on the ITU is due to many factors including hypovolaemia and sepsis. Epidural infusions may be stopped if they are considered to be contributing to hypotension and they are contraindicated in sepsis.

### 6.3.1.3 *Patient-controlled analgesia*

As soon as the patient is able to use a PCA, continuous opiate infusions should be stopped. PCA offers a suitable method of analgesic delivery in a high dependency area. Good analgesia must be achieved by effective PCA use, prior to transfer to the wards.

## References

Dolin SJ, Cashman JN, and Bland JM (2002). Effectiveness of acute postoperative pain management. Evidence from published data. *British Journal of Anaesthesia*, **89**, 409–29.

Eugene R and Viscusi MD (2004). Patient-controlled transdermal fentanyl hydrochloride vs intravenous morphine pump for postoperative pain. *JAMA*, **91**, 1333–41.

Jin F and Chug F (2001). Multimodal analgesia for postoperative pain. *Journal of Clinical Anaesthesia*, **13**, 524–39.

Perkins FM and Kehlet H (2000). Chronic pain as an outcome of surgery. A review of predictive factors. *Anesthesiology*, **93**, 1123.

Royal College of Anaesthetists. (1998). RCA guidelines for the use of NSAIDs in perioperative period. RCA, Oxford, UK.

Royal College of Surgeons of England, College of Anaesthetists (1990). Report of the working party on pain after surgery. Rpyal College of Surgeons/College of Anaesthetists, London, UK..

# Chapter 7

# Day surgery analgesia

Damon Kamming

## Key points

- Seventy-five per cent of all elective surgery will soon be day surgery.
- Thirty to fifty per cent of the patients do not take post discharge analgesia 'around the clock' regularly as instructed.
- Thirty per cent of the patients experience moderate to severe pain post discharge as a result of only taking analgesia 'as required' after day surgery.
- Patient education in preassessment clinic (PAC) is vital to ensure that patients understand day surgery analgesia management.
- Proactive pre-emptive and multimodal analgesia utilizing regional anaesthesia reduce opioid-related side effects and enable discharge home.
- Post discharge regular multimodal analgesia is key to achieving goal of mild post discharge pain scores.
- Patient follow up is vital for audit and ensuring quality clinical care.

## 7.1 Introduction

The Department of Health has set a target of 75% of elective surgery being undertaken as day surgery. The audit commission has estimated that if surgeons default suitable surgery for day surgery, there is a potential to release half a million inpatient bed days a year across the National Health Service (NHS). Admitting surgical patients unnecessarily into hospital overnight costs the NHS £1 billion a year and deprives patients of the comfort of their homes and the company of their family. The development of short-acting, rapidly eliminated anaesthetic drugs with minimal side effects combined with minimal invasive surgery improves the speed of recovery and reduces the need for overnight hospital admission. Instead of asking 'why day surgery?' we are now asking 'why not day surgery?' Evidence demonstrates that day surgery is effective, efficient, and safe.

### 7.1.1 Pain is the problem

Evidence suggests that between 30% and 45% of day surgery patients experience moderate to severe pain at home after discharge. Pain has adverse associated physiological sequelae, delays surgical healing, and is a risk factor for the development of chronic pain. Uncontrolled pain after day surgery can result in overnight admission with its financial implications, delay return to work with its economical implications, can increase the demand on the family with its social implications, and may put pressure on primary care services with its resource implications. Management of pain after day surgery is a priority for all concerned.

### 7.1.2 Day surgery revolution

Developments in anaesthesia across two centuries have reduced suffering, and optimized perioperative safety and post-operative morbidity in the hospital environment. At the beginning of the 20th century, a Scottish paediatric surgeon, James Nicoll suggested that paediatric patients were better nursed at home by their mothers. This argument can also be made for elderly patients who may benefit from day surgery as long as any chronic disease is stable. In the 21st century, improvements in anaesthetic pharmacology synergize with increasing use of minimally invasive surgery enabling the acceptance of older and sicker patients.

The aim is to move the patient from a state of surgical anaesthesia to street fitness in the shortest possible time with the lowest incidence of side effects. To achieve this a suitable pain management strategy must be given to the patient, which can be managed without further medical input.

Day surgery or ambulatory surgery requires the patient to 'walk' out of hospital. Day surgery analgesia is all about enabling post-operative ambulation, by minimizing the side effects of analgesia, such as sedation dizziness and nausea and vomiting.

## 7.2 Preassessment

At the preassessment clinic (PAC), the empowering process of self-managing post-operative pain begins with a discussion about how this will be managed. A dialogue is established about realistic expectations of post-operative analgesia. Patients are educated that mild pain is an expected and normal response to surgery. Twenty per cent of these patients do worry about experiencing more severe pain at home. But most patients prefer mild pain and minimal side effects and to be at home to no pain but with distressing side effects and an overnight hospital admission. Instructions to take analgesia on a regular basis post-operatively 'around the clock' for at least 3 days need to be reinforced verbally and with an information sheet. This gives the patient time to assimilate the information so they can ask any questions on the day of surgery. This message is re-emphasized at every stage. Inadequate education results in 30–50% of patients' not taking analgesia regularly post discharge and leads to complaints of moderate to severe pain associated with delayed recovery from surgery.

### 7.2.1 Planning anaesthesia

It is important to remember that some post-operative pain can be directly attributed to anaesthetic technique. About 40–85% of young fit healthy patients receiving suxamethonium chloride (succinylcholine) for intubation will complain of severe post-operative myalgia, which will impede mobilization and will increase time to discharge and dissatisfaction for the patient. Using alfentanil or remifentanil as an aid to intubation is a better technique for day surgery. Regional anaesthesia will be discussed independently below.

### 7.2.2 Pre-emptive analgesia

Pre-emptive analgesia implies that giving analgesia before surgery will produce a greater analgesic effect than if given after surgery. Achieving steady-state therapeutic concentrations of analgesics before surgical skin incision has been shown to reduce post-operative pain scores and analgesic requirements in the first 24hr after discharge. The improved analgesic effect may be due to preventing the peripheral and central sensitization caused initially by the surgical skin incision and later by the inflammatory injury. Giving the patient intravenous paracetamol and an intravenous non-steroidal anti-inflammatory drug (NSAID) before skin incision reduces the amount of perioperative opioid required, reducing the associated side effects. Co-administering paracetamol and an NSAID before surgery can result in a 30–40% reduction in opioid analgesic requirement. Local anaesthetics should be injected or infiltrated before skin incision. If patients have a history of chronic pain, cannot tolerate NSAIDs, cannot or will not have regional, then a pre-emptive small dose ketamine (0.1mg/kg) given post induction as a co-analgesic is a method of reducing post-operative pain and reducing opioid requirement without increasing side effects.

Adjuvants are compounds which alone have low analgesic potency but in combination with opioids allow a reduction of opioids for post-operative pain control, reducing the occurrence of side effects. Gabapentin is an anticonvulsant that has proven useful in the treatment of chronic pain. Pre-emptive gabapentin (1.2g) has been used in day surgery and can reduce post-operative opioid requirements; however, it can result in increased post-operative dizziness and sedation that can affect effective ambulation and increase time to discharge.

## 7.3 **Perioperative multimodal analgesia**

Opioid analgesics are the traditional cornerstone of perioperative analgesia but they are commonly associated with nausea, vomiting, sedation, pruritus, respiratory depression, constipation, and urinary hesitancy and retention (all of which can prevent discharge home). Multimodal analgesia refers to the use of more than one mode of action of analgesia to produce effective analgesia through different mechanisms. Multimodal analgesia is key to reducing the overall post-operative side effect profile. If regional anaesthesia or analgesia is not possible, then in addition to intravenous paracetamol and intravenous NSAIDs intravenous opioids will be necessary.

### 7.3.1 **Opioids**

Remifentanil has limited use for day surgery because it provides no post-operative analgesia and can cause acute opioid tolerance intra-operatively causing a paradoxical increase in post-operative pain and opioid consumption. Morphine gives good analgesia but results in a high percentage of patients suffering from nausea and vomiting on mobilizing and limits ambulation, therefore delaying discharge home. In day surgery, fentanyl is the preferred opioid analgesic. Incremental intravenous fentanyl titrated against pulse, blood pressure, and respiratory rate offers a good balance between quick onset (2–4min) and moderate duration of offset (45min). Fentanyl as compared with morphine halves the incidence of nausea and vomiting on the journey home.

### 7.3.2 **Non-steroidal anti-inflammatory drugs**

The Royal College of Anaesthetists have stated that NSAIDs are the analgesic of choice in day surgery. For those patients with no contraindications, they are an essential component of multimodal analgesia. Drugs which occur in both parenteral form and oral form provide the most elegant solution. Intravenous diclofenac perioperatively and oral diclofenac post-operatively is a common pre-operative choice of NSAIDs, or dexketoprofen, which has a more rapid onset of action than diclofenac, and is also available in both intravenous and oral forms.

### 7.3.3 **Paracetamol**

Paracetamol has always been part of multimodal intraoperative analgesia. Paracetamol suppositories may be used, but the introduction of intravenous preparations of paracetamol has allowed its perioperative administration with a 100% bioavailability. It is now a mainstay of day surgery intraoperative analgesia.

### 7.3.4 **Prophylactic multimodal anti-emesis**

When considering analgesia for day surgery, it is also important to consider anti-emesis.

All day surgery patients should be considered as a high risk for post-operative nausea and vomiting (PONV). The incidence is about 30% in most studies and PONV can be minimized by general strategies such as a minimal fluid fasting time of 2hr, perioperative hydration with 20mL/kg of intravenous fluid, avoiding general anaesthesia (GA) and utilizing regional anaesthesia. Where GA is used, avoidance of nitrous oxide is important. Prophylactic perioperative anti-emetics are given; dexamethasone 4–8mg has a number-needed-to-treat of 2 as an anti-emetic and also reduces post-operative pain. Proactive use of intravenous fentanyl rather than morphine in recovery reduces the problems of PONV. Tramadol produces a high incidence of dizziness and related PONV and should be reserved for NSAID-intolerant patients unsuitable for regional anaesthesia. It has the greatest frequency of side effects with substantial patient dissatisfaction. Current guidelines support the use of multimodal anti-emesis with ondanscrton/granisetron combined with dexamethasone for patients at high risk of PONV.

## 7.4 Regional anaesthesia

Regional anaesthesia is ideal for many peripheral day surgical procedures. The choice of technique depends on patient factors and surgical factors. Details of different techniques can be found in standard texts. Regional anaesthesia may be used as the sole anaesthetic or used in combination with GA as appropriate.

The disadvantages of regional techniques include the additional time required to perform and await the onset of the block and the potential risk of neurological complications which requires extra time at the consenting process. The use of ultrasound-guided regional anaesthesia can potentially speed up the process, improve the success rate and reduce the side effects.

### 7.4.1 Upper and lower limb blocks

The use of upper and lower peripheral nerve blocks provides excellent prolonged analgesia with minimal side effects. Arthroscopic shoulder surgery is now performed under an interscalene nerve block either with the patient awake or asleep as the patient prefers. A combination of 10mL of 1% lidocaine with 20mL of 0.25% bupivacaine is used for plexus blocks for day surgery. Studies have demonstrated that without an interscalene nerve block 8% of patients required overnight admission because of severe pain. None of the patients with an interscalene block required admission. A patient with an insensate extremity can be safely discharge home; however, they need to understand the need to take special care of their numb, heavy, weak, blocked limb. These patients will need regular multimodal analgesia up to a week post-operatively. The patient must take maximal prescribed multimodal analgesia 1hr before the anticipated wearing off of the block approximately 18hrs afterwards. Patients are instructed to take oral analgesia 18hrs after the nerve block was established irrespective of whether or not they are in pain at the time.

Physiotherapy is delayed with the use of lower limb plexus blocks especially early static quadriceps contraction. This is integral to achieving the desired early mobilization after arthroscopic anterior cruciate ligament repairs. In arthroscopic surgery, evidence continues to support the use of intra-articular local anaesthetic and intra-articular morphine.

### 7.4.2 Neuroaxial anaesthesia

Spinal anaesthesia remains an option in day surgery. The dose of heavy bupivacaine should be reduced to between 5mg and 10mg (1–2mL) to enable prompt return of reflexes and to reduce the risk of urinary retention. Adding 12.5mcg fentanyl improves the quality of the block. Additional intravenous paracetamol and NSAIDs are given to provide multimodal analgesic cover for when the neuraxial block wears off. Patients should be warned about the associated risks including dural puncture headache and urinary retention.

## 7.5 Post-operative analgesia

### 7.5.1 First stage recovery

Fentanyl boluses of 20mcg to a total of 2–4mcg/kg are effective and easily titratable method of perioperative analgesia that can be continued into first stage recovery. Recovery nursing staff can follow a protocol whereby they will give 20mcg boluses of fentanyl every 5min until the pain is described as mild. At this point, the patient is given an oral longer-acting opioid such as dihydrocodeine.

### 7.5.2 Second stage recovery—ward

When the patient is alert and orientated, discharge to the ward area and preparation for discharge is the next stage.

Crews (2002) has published an analgesic ladder for multimodal post-operative pain management for ambulatory surgical procedures based on the World Health Organization (WHO) analgesic ladder for cancer pain management.

Therapy for each patient begins at Step 1, with medications or regional anaesthetic interventions considered in subsequent steps in response to increased pain intensity (see Table 7.1) for multimodal analgesia is be proactive rather than reactive.

### 7.5.3 Discharge analgesia

About 30% of day surgery patients have moderate to severe pain after discharge home. This is often worse on the second post-operative

| Table 7.1 Day surgery analgesic ladder |
| --- |
| **Step 1** |
| • Minor surgical procedures |
|     • Paracetamol |
|     • NSAIDs |
|     • Local anaesthetic infiltration |
| **Step 2** |
| • Moderate surgical procedures |
|     • Step 1 therapy |
|     • + Intermittent boluses of fentanyl |
| **Step 3** |
| • Major surgery or patients expected to have high post-operative analgesic requirements |
|     • Step 2 therapy |
|     • + Plexus block or other major peripheral block |
|     • + Consider sustained release opiates |

day as they start to mobilize. It is essential, therefore, that instructions for analgesia are re-enforced with the patient before discharge. Anxieties about the taking of regular analgesia, such as delayed healing, are alleviated. A follow up phone call post discharge can be used to audit effectiveness of treatment. Effective post discharge analgesia must be safe, with minimal side effects, and be easily understood and managed at home up to a week post-operatively. The patient should be reminded that they must take the analgesia dispensed regularly as prescribed for at least the first 3 days depending on the surgery. More complex surgery will require regular analgesia for at least a week post-operatively.

In the future, post discharge patient-controlled transdermal, intra-nasal analgesia, and patient-controlled local anaesthesia with safe disposable infusion systems are likely to become available.

### 7.5.4 Patient satisfaction

Patient satisfaction with pain management is complex and subject to cultural and individual variables. Surveys suggest that 50% of patients would 'tolerate' pain after discharge from hospital rather than 'complain' about it to their caregivers. Pain is ranked in the top three most undesirable outcomes after day surgery. Patient's reports of satisfaction with their post-operative pain management may not necessarily reflect well-controlled pain during their recovery. Audit by telephone of clarity of instructions and pain control given to the patient post discharge is a tool to close the audit loop and an effective mechanism for extending quality of patient care. The expansion of day surgery depends on excellent self-management of post-operative pain at home without relying on primary care or accident and emergency.

The discharge criteria used to discharge day surgery patients home is the post-anaesthetic discharge scoring system (PADSS) and one of the components of this is pain being sufficiently controlled with oral analgesia before discharge.

## 7.6 Conclusions

Day surgery encourages people to ambulate and empowers them to manage their own pain control. In order to achieve this, we need to educate the patient preoperatively and provide them with high-quality advice about pain management post discharge. Day Surgery and Pain Medicine are specialities where there is continuation of care into the community. Collaboration between the two specialities can achieve great results for day surgery patients. As day surgery embraces more complex and challenging patients and procedures, we need to ensure that the quality of care does not suffer and that the patient remains the prime focus of our endeavours both in hospital but now more importantly at home as well.

## References

Crews JC (2002). Multi-modal pain management strategies for office based and ambulatory procedures. *JAMA*, **288**, 629–32.

Gan TJ, Meyer T, Apfel CC, *et al.* (2003). Consensus guidelines for managing postoperative nausea and vomiting. *Anesthesia & Analgesia*, **97**, 62–71.

Klein SM, Bergh A, Steele SM, *et al.* (2005). Peripheral nerve block techniques for ambulatory surgery. *Anesthesia & Analgesia*, **101**, 1663–76.

McGrath B, Elgendy H, Chung F, *et al.* (2004). Thirty percent of patients have moderate to severe pain 24hr after ambulatory surgery: a survey of 5,703 patients. *Canadian Journal of Anaesthesia*, **51**, 886–91.

Rawal N (2001). Analgesia for day-case surgery. *British Journal of Anaesthesia*, **87**, 73–87.

Smith I, Cooke T, Jackson I, and Fitzpatrick R (2006). Rising to the challenges of achieving day surgery targets. *Anaesthesia*, **61**, 1191–9.

White PF (2005). The changing role of non-opioid analgesic techniques in the management of postoperative pain. *Anesthesia & Analgesia*, **101**, S5–22.

# Chapter 8

# Trauma pain and procedural pain: prevention of chronic pain following acute trauma

Brigitta Brandner and Johan Emmanuel

### Key points

- Opioid analgesics should be used with extreme cautions in the self-ventilating head injured patient.
- Gastric emptying ceases after trauma. This will limit the efficacy of oral analgesics.
- Epidural analgesia has been shown to be an independent predictor of decreased morbidity and mortality in thoracic trauma.
- Femoral nerve block is as effective as intravenous morphine in femoral shaft fractures.
- Short-term non-steroidal anti-inflammatory drug use has no proven deleterious effects in humans, and should be part of multimodal management.
- Trauma is a risk factor for complex regional pain syndrome. Prevention should be aimed at early graded mobilizations with adequate pain relief.
- Post-amputation pain encompasses stump pain (nociceptive and neuropathic), and phantom limb pain.

## 8.1 Acute pain after trauma

The management of the trauma patient is set out in the Advanced Trauma and Life Support manual, with a framework that includes rigorous assessment, and simultaneous resuscitation. This framework will ensure that no life-threatening injuries are missed. However, inadequate management of pain in the trauma patient is a common problem. Concerns over cardiovascular and respiratory compromise, and masking of clinical signs leave the patient distressed with pain.

The distressed patient in pain can lead to problems by himself, with the lack of cooperation making treatment more complicated, and placing undue stress on the body.

## 8.1.1 Pathophysiological changes in trauma

### 8.1.1.1 *Head injury*

Following head injury, there are two distinct periods: a primary insult, the result of mechanical forces upon the soft tissues; and a secondary insult, the consequence of physiological insults such as ischaemia and reperfusion upon the damaged areas of brain. The early management is therefore directed towards minimizing the secondary insult.

Autoregulation of the cerebral vasculature is abolished in traumatic brain injury and maintenance of adequate oxygenation and avoidance of hypercapnia is important. Therefore, opioid analgesics must be used with caution in this situation.

### 8.1.1.2 *Thoracic injury*

Blunt chest trauma is a significant preventable cause of death in trauma patients. Tissue hypoxia may be due to hypovolaemia, pneumothorax, cardiac injury, or areas of ventilation/perfusion mismatch. Hypercarbia can also develop due to mechanical causes such as flail segments or reduced ventilation due to pain. In addition, pain will also limit clearance of secretions, thus further compounding the problem. The appropriate analgesic management is essential in this group of patients to reduce morbidity and mortality.

### 8.1.1.3 *Circulatory*

Hypovolaemia activates compensatory mechanisms, with sympathetically mediated arterial and venoconstriction. In an attempt to maintain perfusion to vital organs (brain, heart, kidney), blood supply is redirected away form skin and subcutaneous tissues, thus making the bioavailability of intramuscular injections unreliable.

### 8.1.1.4 *Gastric physiology*

Peristaltic waves sweep from the cardia to pylorus at a rate of 3/min. The rate of gastric emptying is proportional to the volume of stomach contents, with approximately 2% of the contents emptied into the duodenum per minute. There are many conditions known to decrease gastric emptying, opioid analgesics being but one; however, importantly in trauma gastric emptying virtually ceases. This will have an impact when considering the use of oral analgesics.

## 8.2 **Pain management in the pre-hospital setting**

To those attending to these patients, this can be the most challenging environment. The variation in the level of training of responders, availability of medication, equipment, and the setting mean that a limited amount of analgesic options are available. Intravenous morphine is available as the analgesic of choice; however, sometimes intravenous access is not possible, and concerns about respiratory depression, sedation, and airway protection mean that other analgesics should be considered. Listed in the following paragraphs are three agents that will have specific benefits in this environment.

### 8.2.1 **Oral transmucosal fentanyl**

An opioid analgesic that is in common use in the hospital setting, recent interest has centred in its use to treat combat victims in the field. Its high-lipid solubility make it the only opioid suitable for transmucosal absorption.

It is available in 200–1600mcg strengths, with an onset of 5min, a peak effect at 20–40min, and a duration of 3hr, although this can increase up to 5hr due to the impaired gastric emptying in trauma patients.

Common to all opioids dose-related side effects include somnolence, nausea, vomiting, and pruritus. Factors that will reduce its transmucosal absorption include reduced saliva, ingestion of liquids that reduce oral pH (coffee, cola, fruit juices), and active chewing of the lozenge.

### 8.2.2 **Intranasal ketamine**

An NMDA receptor antagonist with potent analgesic and sedative properties. Commonly used intravenously or intramuscularly, recent interest has been focused on its intranasal application. Side effects include dizziness, nausea, increased secretions, and hallucinations. Sympathetic stimulation make it unsuitable for those with ischaemic heart disease and hypertension, and increasing intracranial pressure and intraocular pressure make it unsuitable for those with head injury or ocular damage.

In higher doses ketamine, 2mg/kg intravenously or 10mg/kg intramuscularly, produces dissociative anaesthesia. Airway reflexes are maintained, and its bronchodilator and cardiovascular stability make ketamine a useful drug in the unstable patient. The intranasal dose is 2.5–10mg. Higher doses of up to 50mg were effective but had a higher incidence of side effects.

### 8.2.3 Entonox®

Entonox® is the trade name given to a 50:50 mixture of oxygen and nitrous oxide. Nitrous oxide is an anaesthetic gas with significant analgesic properties that has a predictable onset and offset action. It is a gas mixture at normal temperatures stored in a blue cylinder with white shoulders. Administered as an inhalation agent, careful storage is needed as liquefaction and separation of the two components may occur at temperatures of −7°C. It causes minimal cardiovascular or respiratory depression, however, is contraindicated in pneumothoraces as it diffuses into air-filled spaces. Increasing intracranial pressure also limits its use in head injury patients.

## 8.3 Pain management of blunt thoracic trauma

The mortality and morbidity associated with blunt thoracic trauma is significant. Rib fractures are common and have been detected in up to two thirds of chest trauma. Isolated rib fractures are common in the elderly, and can result in a mortality of 8%. The principle cause of this morbidity and mortality is respiratory complications. In one study, 6% of patients with blunt thoracic trauma died, with approximately half of these deaths attributed to secondary respiratory complications. Furthermore, inadequate pain management can lead to increased intensive care unit and ventilator usage.

The current management principles focus on pain relief, chest physiotherapy, and mobilization.

### 8.3.1 Analgesic modalities

#### 8.3.1.1 *Intravenous opioids*

The most common form of analgesic used in clinical practice. Patient-controlled analgesia involves the administration of an intermittent intravenous dose of opioid delivered by the patient. It is easy to administer, without the need of invasive procedures, and not involving specialized personnel. The disadvantages are common to all opioids: nausea, sedation, and respiratory depression.

#### 8.3.1.2 *Epidural analgesia*

Epidural analgesia has been shown to be an independent predictor of decreased morbidity and mortality in thoracic trauma. It involves the administration of local anaesthetic with or without opioid into the epidural space by the introduction of a catheter by specialist medical personnel. The advantages are lack of sedation enabling cooperation with physiotherapy, improved respiratory function, and bilateral analgesic effects. As with all invasive procedures, patients must be informed of the risks (failure, hypotension, dural puncture, spinal cord and nerve injury, infection, and haematoma), and give informed consent. Epidural narcotics can cause nausea and vomiting, urinary retention, and pruritus. Contraindications include patient refusal, allergy to local anaesthetic, coagulation abnormalities, and skin infection at the desired site. Specialist nursing is needed to monitor the somatic and sympathetic effects of the epidural.

### 8.3.1.3 *Thoracic paravertebral block*

Thoracic paravertebral block involves the administration of local anaesthetic in close proximity to thoracic vertebrae. It provides a unilateral somatic and sympathetic block that extends over multiple dermatomes. Similar to epidural analgesia, a catheter can be inserted to provide continuous pain relief. It is thought to be technically easier than an epidural catheter; however, its main advantages are reduced risk of spinal cord injury and unilateral sympathetic blockade. The most common complications are vascular puncture and pneumothorax.

### 8.3.1.4 *Intrapleural analgesia*

This involves the administration of local anaesthetic into the pleural space. It produces unilateral intercostal blocks across multiple dermatomes by diffusion across the parietal pleura. Similar to thoracic paravertebral block, it provides a unilateral blockade; therefore, reducing the sympathetic side effects common with epidural analgesia. Local anaesthetic can affect diaphragmatic function if diffusion travels inferiorly, and patient position, blood in the pleural space, and a chest drain will reduce the effectiveness.

### 8.3.1.5 *Intercostal nerve blockade*

Involves the insertion of local anaesthetic into the posterior component of the intercostal space. Because of the overlap of the intercostal nerves, blocks will have to be given above, below, and at the level of the fractured rib. It is a relatively easy technique; however, the effect lasts only with upper 6hr, so multiple injection will be needed. In addition, palpation of the ribs is needed to identify landmarks, which may be painful, and the scapula obstructs any attempts at the upper ribs.

## 8.4 Regional techniques for femoral fractures

Peripheral nerve block provides distinct benefits in this group of patients. Femoral nerve blockade is as quick and effective as intravenous morphine, avoids opioid side effects, which are problematic in the elderly, and enables the patients to sit up quickly.

Epidural analgesia has been shown to be particularly useful in high-risk cardiac patients with fractured neck of femurs when sited preoperatively. Whilst epidural analgesia should be performed by an anaesthetist, nerve blockade is a relatively simple procedure, and is being employed by emergency doctors, and indeed by some trained nurses. Much of the reluctance to insert peripheral nerve blockade preoperatively is concerned with the lack of training and equipment and perceived risk.

Two peripheral nerve blocks for femoral fractures are described here. Some general considerations must be made before embarking on a peripheral nerve block. Facilities for resuscitation should be available, the patient should be consented for the procedure, and aseptic techniques should be employed. Absolute contraindications include patient refusal, infection, or haematoma in the vicinity of the puncture site and allergy.

## 8.4.1 Femoral nerve block

Also described as the three-in-one block because of the theory that one injection blocks three nerves (femoral, obturator, and lateral femoral cutaneous nerves).

### 8.4.1.1 *Anatomy*

The femoral nerve is the largest branch of the lumbar plexus. It descends in the fibres of the psoas muscle. It emerges from under the inguinal ligament lateral to the femoral artery.

### 8.4.1.2 *Landmarks*

- Femoral artery
- Inguinal ligament—line between anterior superior iliac spine and pubic tubercle.

### 8.4.1.3 *Equipment*

- Assistant
- Peripheral nerve stimulator with stimulating needle
- Syringe
- Local anaesthetic.

### 8.4.1.4 *Method*

The patient is positioned on their back with legs slightly spread apart. The foot of the leg to be anaesthetized should be turned slightly to the outside. The puncture site is approximately 1.5cm lateral to the femoral artery, 2cm below the inguinal ligament.

A small skin wheal is raised with lidocaine (*note*—not too deep otherwise stimulation of femoral nerve will be affected).

The stimulation needle is inserted at an angle of 30% to skin, and advanced cranially.

Stimulation of the rectus muscle of the thigh (shown by patella movement) is the indication that the femoral nerve is close.

The nerve stimulator current is then lowered (0.2–0.5mA) to obtain the best motor response.

Before injecting the local anaesthetic, aspiration should be performed initially, and after each 5mL of solution a finger placed beneath the puncture site will promote spread in a cranial direction.

### 8.4.2 Fascia iliacus nerve block

#### 8.4.2.1 *Anatomy*

The femoral nerve passes under the inguinal ligament, and in the femoral crease area it is covered by the fascia iliacus and separated from the femoral artery and vein by a portion of the psoas muscle and iliopectineal ligament. The nerve lies beneath two fascial planes: the fascia lata and the fascia iliacus. As this is sheath block, the needle can be inserted away from the neurovascular bundle, removing the needle for nerve stimulation, and the risk of neurovascular injury.

#### 8.4.2.2 *Landmarks*

- Anterior superior iliac spine
- Pubic tubercle
- Divide the line from the anterior superior iliac spine and pubic tubercle into equal thirds.
- The entry site is 1cm inferior to the junction of the lateral one-third to the medial two thirds.

#### 8.4.2.3 *Equipment*

- Blunt-tipped needle
- Syringe
- Local anaesthetic: volume 0.3–0.5mL/kg.

#### 8.4.2.4 *Method*

Raise a small skin wheal with lidocaine. Insert the blunt-tipped needle, and insert until two distinct pops are felt (these represent the two fascial layers). Attach the syringe, and after aspiration deposit the local anaesthetic.

## 8.5 Analgesia for distal forearm fracture

Fractures of the distal forearm bones, especially Colles' fracture, are a frequent presentation to the emergency department. The decision to manipulate is dependent on multiple factors, age, functional need, and displacement angulation. The ability to provide analgesia for the manipulation can reduce the need for sedation, and even general anaesthesia. Below will be described two techniques for Colles' fracture management. Bier block has been shown to provide better analgesia, with less need for remanipulation, and therefore better anatomical restoration. There have been no reports of toxicity with prilocaine intravenous regional anaesthesia when used appropriately. Indeed with haematoma blockade, systemic absorption of local anaesthetic doses occur and there is a increased risk of carpal tunnel syndrome, and ensuing median nerve neuropathy.

### 8.5.1 Intravenous regional anaesthesia (Bier block)

Originally described by Bier in 1908, this technique involves the intravenous administration of local anaesthetic into an exsanguinated limb, with a tourniquet to prevent proximal spread. This will provide analgesia for operative procedure less than 60min duration. It is contraindicated in severe Raynaud's disease, sickle cell disease, and crush injury to the limb. Complications are due to leakage of local anaesthetic past the cuff into systemic circulation: dizziness, nausea, vomiting, tinnitus, perioral tingling, muscle twitching, loss of consciousness, and convulsions.

#### 8.5.1.1 *Equipment*

- Two medical personnel with resuscitation facilities available
- Blood pressure and ECG monitoring
- Two intravenous cannulae—one in the affected limb and one at another site
- Single or double cuff tourniquet
- Local anaesthetic—40mL of 0.5% prilocaine (70kg adult).

#### 8.5.1.2 *Method*

Monitoring is attached and cannulae inserted in the affected arm, and in the unaffected arm for resuscitation if necessary. The affected limb is exsanguinated using an Eschmarch bandage or by elevating the arm whilst occluding brachial artery. The tourniquet is inflated to 50–100mg greater than patient's systolic pressure, and the local anaesthetic is slowly injected into the affected limb. The tourniquet must remain inflated for a minimum of 20min.

### 8.5.2 Haematoma block

This consists of injection of local anaesthetic into the fracture site. It is simple to perform with no specialized equipment needed. The complications are infection risk and median nerve neuropathy due to increased carpal tunnel pressure.

#### 8.5.2.1 *Equipment*

- Needle and syringe
- Local anaesthetic—10mL of 1% lidocaine.

#### 8.5.2.2 *Method*

- Insert needle into fracture site
- Inject local anaesthetic.

## 8.6 **Compartment syndrome**

This represents an orthopaedic emergency. The musculoskeletal structure of limbs consists of isolated compartments created by inelastic fascial sheets.

Compartment syndrome occurs when the pressure in one or more of the compartments increases dramatically and limits tissue perfusion causing ischaemic necrosis. This condition can occur with increase in the contents of the compartment or anything that limits distension of the compartment.

It is more common in lower leg and forearm, although can occur in hand, foot, and upper parts of the limbs. Closed tibial fractures are the most common cause; however, it can occur with open fractures. Contrary to the belief, it does not have to be associated with bony injuries.

### 8.6.1 **Pathophysiology**

Increasing compartment pressure causes lymphatic and venous obstruction, further increasing compartment pressure. Tissue perfusion is compromised leading to tissue ischaemia with the release of vasoactive substances. Increase in endothelial permeability and interstitial oedema lead to worsening tissue perfusion. Tissue acidosis ensues with muscle breakdown and myoglobin released, and nerve function is impaired.

### 8.6.2 **Diagnosis**

The diagnosis is predominantly clinical looking for Pain/Pallor/absent Pulse/Paresis; however, pallor and absent pulse are rarely present, and paresis is a late sign. A more reliable indicator is to look for pain out of proportion to injury especially with passive stretch, a palpable tense extremity compared with uninjured limb, and compartment pressure >30mmHg with normal blood pressure (if available).

### 8.6.3 **Treatment**

The surgical will be a fasciotomy; however, it should not be forgotten that these patients may be systemically unwell due to acidosis and renal dysfunction.

### 8.6.4 **Regional anaesthesia and compartment syndrome**

As regional anaesthetic techniques can mask pain (an important diagnostic tool), the clinician must weigh risk to benefit before undertaking the nerve blockade. The reduced incidence of compartment syndrome in the upper leg is thought to be related to the ability of the large muscle bulk to dissipate the force of direct trauma. There has been no evidence that femoral nerve block can delay compartment syndrome in femoral shaft fractures.

## 8.7 Non-steroidal anti-inflammatory drugs and bone healing

Non-steroidal anti-inflammatory drugs (NSAIDs) exert their analgesic effects by inhibiting the production of prostaglandins in the spinal cord and periphery. Prostaglandins are important mediators in bone metabolism, favouring bone formation, and therefore NSAIDs should be deleterious in bone healing.

However, disagreement still exists as to whether this is the correct mechanism through which NSAIDs affect bone healing.

### 8.7.1 Animal studies

Most studies in animals have demonstrated delayed fracture healing. In these studies, NSAIDs were administered over several weeks to months at doses greater than those used in normal clinical practice.

These effects are generally dose dependent and reversible.

There is considerable debate as to which animal model equates to human experience.

### 8.7.2 Human studies

Human studies have shown a mixture of results. However,

- Short-term post-operative administration seems to have no significant effects on bone healing. In spinal fusion surgery, NSAIDs showed additional benefit for chronic donor site pain
- Human studies have failed to demonstrate any deleterious effect on bone density or any increase in fracture risk
- Indometacin should be used with caution in patients with hip replacement and concomitant long-bone fractures, and may cause heterotrophic bone formation after spinal cord injury
- NSAIDs have a proven benefit in the multimodal management of pain in the orthopaedic patient. Whilst there is a theoretical risk, there is no firm evidence that short-term administration of NSAID causes harm.

## 8.8 Acute to chronic pain

The progression from acute to chronic pain is an important area of study, the pathophysiology is being investigated and greater attempts are being made to limit the progression to chronic pain states. Acute pain serves a biological function, to prevent further tissue damage, but chronic pain continues beyond the natural healing process. In addition with chronic pain states, one must consider the psychosocial elements when treating. Trauma is associated with chronic pain states, chronic pain syndrome, post-amputation pain syndrome, and chronic whiplash injury.

### 8.8.1 **Complex regional pain syndrome**

Complex regional pain syndromes (CRPS) encompass a variety of chronic pain conditions with pain associated with vasomotor changes. These syndromes were classified by the International Association or the Study of Pain (IASP) in 1994 into reflex sympathetic dystrophy (CRPS type 1), causalgia, and post-traumatic neuralgia (CRPS type 2).

#### 8.8.1.1 *Diagnostic criteria IASP–CRPS type 1*

- The presence of an initiating noxious event or a cause of immobilization
- Continuing pain, allodynia, or hyperalgesia disproportionate to any inciting event
- Evidence at some time of oedema, changes in skin blood flow, or abnormal sudomotor activity in the area of pain
- Exclusion of other conditions that would account for the pain and dysfunction
- CRPS type 2 is differentiated by the presence of nerve injury as the primary mechanism.

Trauma is a common aetiology in the development of CRPS, with sprains/strains and fractures accounting for 45% in one study of presentations with CRPS to a tertiary pain clinic. Although much of the pathophysiology of the condition remains to be elucidated, immobilization and disuse are important risk factors, and early graded mobilization should be encouraged. Surgical management has been shown to worsen the condition. Interest in post-surgical CRPS has focused on the pre-emptive multimodal analgesic techniques with a role for preoperative sympathetic blockade in conjunction with physical therapy and rehabilitation. Pharmacological therapies using vitamin C and ketanserin (a serotonin type 2 receptor antagonist) have also shown promise.

If untreated, this condition will progress to disability; therefore, once diagnosed a multidisciplinary approach focusing on physical therapy to restore function to the affected limb, and manage the pain with pharmacotherapy, interventions, and behavioural therapy if indicated.

### 8.8.2 **Post-amputation pain syndrome**

Pain syndromes after amputation include stump pain and phantom limb pain.

*Stump pain* usually commences in the early post-amputation period and subsides over time as tissue healing occurs. However in 5–10%, this pain persists, interfering with the rehabilitation period. In addition, it has been noticed that there is a higher prevalence of phantom limb pain co-existing with those who have stump pain.

Nociceptive stump pain originates from the local structures within the stump and management should be directed to look for causes such as vascular insufficiency, badly fitting prosthesis, adherent scars, skin irritation, etc.

Neuromata within the stump can give rise to neuropathic pain. Surgical removal of these is not conclusive due to regrowth of the neuromata, and so local anaesthetic injections, and pharmacological treatments should be considered.

The mechanisms of *phantom limb pain* have not been completely elucidated with both peripheral and central dysfunction implicated. Phantom limb sensation can also exist but this is not painful. The occurrence of phantom limb pain is independent of age, gender, and level of amputation, reason for amputation. Stump pain, pre-amputation pain and non-painful sensations are recognized as predictors; however, this is not consistent. In addition to the usual therapies for chronic pain, mirror box therapy has been used in this field.

### 8.8.3 **Whiplash**

Whiplash is an acceleration–deceleration injury to the neck commonly a result of a rear end impact. The principal symptoms are of neck, head, and shoulder pain that are aggravated by movement. Muscle spasms of the scalene muscles may be responsible for some of the neurological symptoms referred to the arms. It is now thought that the primary pathology is an arthritic process within the cervical facet joints. Spontaneous remission is unlikely after 3 months, and often ongoing litigation issues obscures their evaluation and treatment by clinicians.

As in most chronic pain conditions, it is important to recognize the psychosocial impact, and recognize that these patients will demonstrate illness behaviour.

Therefore, prevention should be to educate these patients that their injury and pain is benign self-limiting problem. Collars, rest, and negative attitudes and beliefs delay recovery and contribute to chronicity.

## References

Allen G, Galer BS, and Schwartz L (1999). Epidemiology of complex regional pain syndrome: a retrospective chart review of 134 patients. *Pain*, **80**, 539–44.

Bandolier (2004). *NSAIDS, COXIBS, Smoking and Bone*. Bandolier, Oxford.

Curran N and Bradner B (2005). Chronic pain following trauma. *Trauma*, **7**, 123–31.

Karagiannis G (2005). Best evidence topic report. No evidence found that a femoral nerve block in cases of femoral shaft fractures can delay the diagnosis of compartment syndrome. *Emergency Medical Journal*, **22**, 814.

Kotwal RS, O'Connor KC, Johnson TR, et al. (2004). A novel pain management strategy for combat casualty care. *Annals of Emergency Medicine*, **44**, 121–7.

Matot I, Oppenheim-Eden A, Ratrot R, et al. (2003). Pre-operative cardiac events in elderly patients randomized to epidural or conventional analgesia. *Anaesthesiology*, **98**, 156–63.

Meinig RP, Quick A, and Lobmeyer L (1989). Plasma lidocaine levels following hematoma block for distal radius fractures. *Journal of Orthopaedic Trauma*, **3**, 187–91.

Merskey H and Bogduk N (eds) (1994). *Classification of Chronic Pain: Description of Chronic Pain Syndromes and Definition of Pain Terms*, 2nd edn. IASP Press, Seattle, WA, pp. 40–3.

Simon BJ, Cushman J, Barraco R, et al. (2005). Pain management guidelines for blunt thoracic trauma. *The Journal of Trauma: Injury, Infection and Critical Care*, **59**, 1256–67.

Wardrope J, Flowers M, and Wilson DH (1985). Comparison of local anaesthetic techniques in the reduction of Colle's fractures. *Archives of Emergency Medicine*, **2**, 67–72.

Wisner DH (1990). A stepwise logistic regression analysis of factors affecting morbidity and mortality after thoracic trauma: effect of epidural analgesia. *Journal of Trauma: Injury, Infection and Critical Care*, **30**, 799–805; discussion 795–804.

## Chapter 9

# Treatment of pain in burns patients

Edward Welechew

### Key points

- Pain from burns has three components: background, breakthrough, and procedural pain.
- Central sensitization is an important component of the ongoing pain.
- Early management of pain, prior to the arrival at hospital is essential.
- Multimodal treatment including opiates will be necessary and psychological support is key.
- Procedural pain is of high intensity and short duration, and will require a combination of pharmacological and non-pharmacological methods of analgesia.
- Central sensitization and opiate tolerance are common problems in burns patients.

## 9.1 The pathophysiology of burn pain

A burn occurs when skin is exposed to excessive heat, electricity, or corrosive chemicals. Burns are classified by the degree of tissue damage (see Table 9.1).

An individual patient who has extensive burns may have areas of skin that are damaged to a different degree.

The initial injury produces primary hyperalgesia due to damage to nociceptor endings in the dermis and epidermis. Patients with extensive burns also develop secondary hyperalgesia and allodynia, this may be a result of repeated mechanical stimulation due to multiple changes of dressings. Wind up is also part of the phenomena, and burns patients go on having pain, which may increase, during the entire period of treatment and healing.

Inadequate pain management is detrimental and may increase the incidence of post-traumatic stress disorder.

| Table 9.1 Classification of burns | | |
|---|---|---|
| Type of burn | Level of burn | Signs and symptoms |
| First degree | Epidermis | Pain and redness |
| Second degree | Epidermis and dermis | Pain, redness, blistering and ooze |
| Third degree | All layers + underlying muscle tendons and bone | Pale, charred, leaking fluid, no sensation |

### 9.1.1 The nature of pain after burn injury

Pain after burns has three major components: background, breakthrough, and procedural pain, with features of central sensitization to pain appearing as increasingly troublesome complications a few days after the initial burn.

Background pain is not constant but varies during the patient's day. With constant levels of analgesic, there will be periods of breakthrough pain. The analgesic regime, therefore, needs to have both a constant background and a variable element with a rapid onset and potentially short duration.

Procedural pain is of high intensity and of short to medium duration depending on the procedure.

Central sensitization to pain not only amplifies it, but also may widen the painful site beyond the margins of the burn. It may also turn innocuous stimuli at undamaged sites into painful ones.

## 9.2 Pre-hospital and early pain management of the acutely burnt patient

### 9.2.1 Non-pharmacological methods

There are a variety of physical methods to reduce the pain of a burn, which include:

- Cooling, which is often done with cold water
- Wrapping the damaged area in cling film, this helps the pain, and avoids contamination of the burn
- Immobilizing the affected area, avoiding flexion, and minimizing the pressure on the burn also help avoid pain
- Reassurance and compassion for the patient who may be confused, frightened, and distressed.

### 9.2.2 Drugs

*Nitrous oxide in 50% oxygen* (*Entonox®*) delivered by mask using a demand system has a powerful analgesic and sedative effect with a rapid onset and short duration. This is available in cylinders on most ambulances and in Accident and Emergency Departments in Britain.

If the patient is suffering from inhalation injury or carbon monoxide poisoning, 100% oxygen may be needed instead.

*Titration of intravenous opiates directly against the patient's pain.* This is the mainstay of early hospital analgesic management. The subcutaneous and intramuscular routes may be unreliable at this stage because of vasoconstriction whilst the oral route may be ineffective, because of delayed gastric emptying.

Patients with more extensive burns will need resuscitation with intravenous fluids, over 1–2 days. During this period, major shifts in body fluids make maintenance of a constant plasma level of analgesic difficult. Intravenous patient-controlled analgesia (PCA) morphine may be helpful, but more commonly constant infusions of morphine are used—with close supervision and frequent adjustment.

## 9.3 Post-resuscitation management of background and breakthrough pain

### 9.3.1 Intravenous or intramuscular PCA

This is valuable because it can provide both background analgesia with a constant infusion of analgesic and patient-controlled supplements to meet the variable increases in pain due to breakthrough. However, many of these patients may be incapacitated by burnt hands, making operation of PCA buttons difficult. If the handset is taped to the end of the bed or a cot side, it can be pushed with a foot or an elbow.

### 9.3.2 Nurse-controlled infusions

Where greater levels of observation and intervention are possible, nurse-controlled infusions of opiate may be used to deal with background pain and nurse-administered intravenous bolus doses used for breakthrough. This requires nurse training and accreditation in pain assessment and the intravenous administration of opiates.

### 9.3.3 Oral analgesics

Drugs given orally may not be absorbed during the first few days after a burn because of delayed gastric emptying. When enteral nutrition starts—often via a nasogastric or nasojejunal tube, analgesics may be given as liquid, syrup, or suspensions down the tube. Unless contraindicated, oral analgesics should be used as soon as possible to reduce dependence on venous access.

*Oral morphine preparations* or methadone may be used regularly for background pain when the patient is able to take them. Methadone need only be given once or twice daily because of its longer duration.

### 9.3.3.1 *Paracetamol*

Paracetamol is not only analgesic but also antipyretic and helps control the pyrexia commonly seen in burns patients. It can be given orally, rectally, and intravenously. Regular dosing with the intravenous form will lead to significantly higher plasma levels than the same doses given orally and caution should be used in patients with low glutathione levels or reduced hepatic function as hepatic toxicity may occur. Paracetamol given intravenously may reduce opiate requirements by up to 33%.

### 9.3.3.2 *Transmucosal fentanyl*

Fentanyl lozenges (Actiq®) are rubbed against the moist mucosa in the mouth, where the fentanyl is rapidly absorbed and may be helpful for breakthrough pain. This technique has a very short duration and so is unsuitable for background pain. The lowest dose 200mcg lozenge should be tried first and the patient should be carefully monitored when using a new dose lozenge for the first time.

### 9.3.3.3 *Non-steroidal anti-inflammatory drugs*

Patients with minor burns (<10% in children and <15% in adults) may find non-steroidal anti-inflammatory drugs helpful as part of a multimodal analgesic regime. Unfortunately, these drugs may increase bleeding from the burn, increase the risk of gastric bleeding, and may exacerbate renal impairment. Their use in pain management for major burns is therefore limited.

### 9.3.4 **Psychological support**

Patients with major burns often have post-traumatic stress syndrome, which may need counselling, reassurance, and other psychological support. It has been shown that post-traumatic stress syndrome has an adverse effect on the patient's pain whilst severe pain increases their psychological morbidity.

Extensive work in America has shown hypnosis and relaxation therapy to be useful in burns patients. During the first few days after major burns, patients appear to be unusually susceptible to hypnotic suggestion. Daily repetition of the induction process, with instruction in relaxation therapy and self-hypnosis, gives high success rates and both reduces anxiety and increases pain tolerance for background and procedural pain.

## 9.4 **Management of procedural pain**

### 9.4.1 **Burns dressing changes**

The dressings over large burns rapidly become soaked in tissue fluids, blood, and pus. These dressings are commonly changed every 2–3 days and the process may cause great pain and distress for the patient.

### 9.4.1.1 *Non-pharmacological methods*

Soaking dressings in warm saline liquefies dried on and adherent secretions allowing the dressings to be removed without painful tethering to the burn. Patients with extensive burns may need to be lowered into a bath full of warm water to minimize the pain of dressings removal. Moving the patient using a hoist may itself cause pain.

### 9.4.1.2 *Hypnosis and relaxation*

Relaxation therapy and self-hypnosis are helpful in reducing the major anxiety component involved in burns dressing pain. Constant verbal reassurance, sympathy, and encouragement are needed throughout the procedures.

*Distraction* by music from headphones or conversation will often reduce discomfort and distress by preventing anticipation of pain and taking the patient's mental focus away from the procedure.

### 9.4.1.3 *Pharmacological methods*

Nitrous oxide in 50% oxygen (*Entonox*®) delivered from premixed cylinders via a demand valve and mask can provide both analgesia and sedation with a rapid onset and short duration. To use this, patients must hold a mask over their nose and mouth firmly enough to make an airtight seal and inspire deeply enough to trigger the demand valve. Small children or confused patients may not be able to cooperate with this system. Patients with burnt hands or arms may not be able to hold on to the mask and patients with burnt faces may not be able to make an airtight seal with the mask against their faces. However, when administered by enthusiastic, trained nurses, this method is very helpful.

Nitrous oxide administered repeatedly for long periods has been shown to cause bone marrow suppression by the inhibition of methionine synthetase. This limits its use to relatively short procedures no more than once daily. Exhaled nitrous oxide may cause a pollution risk for staff. Staff exposure to nitrous oxide would need to be monitored and kept to a minimum.

### 9.4.1.4 *Opiates*

Morphine is commonly used orally or intravenously for both background and procedural pain. Its use for long-term analgesia is well established and it is well known to most staff. Morphine-6-glucuronide is an active major metabolite, which is renally excreted and so may accumulate when renal function is poor.

*Intravenous PCA* with short-acting opiates, such as fentanyl, may be helpful. When used for burns dressings, the programming of the pump will need to be changed to allow a larger than usual bolus dose and a shorter interval than is used for either background pain or postoperative pain. A bolus dose of 50mcg and a lockout of 3min is often needed for 'normal' adults. There is obviously a risk of respiratory depression when opiates are used in this way and a trained nurse or doctor should be allocated to monitor the patient's condition during the procedure and afterwards. If excessive sedation or respiratory depression occurs, the PCA button must be removed from the patient immediately. Verbal encouragement to breath deeply is usually all that is required. Manual ventilation of the patient with oxygen via a face mask and bag, and valve may be needed for a few minutes and the opiate reversal agent *naloxone* should be available to give intravenously if the patient does not respond sufficiently.

*Pethidine* is shorter acting than morphine and forms norpethidine as an active metabolite, which is excreted from the kidneys. Norpethidine is toxic, causing a potentially lethal mixture of excitation and depression which may be very difficult to treat.

*Ketamine* is an NMDA-blocking agent with powerful analgesic and anaesthetic properties. It may be used intravenously or intramuscularly to produce analgesia and sedation for burn dressings in both adults and children. As it is an anaesthetic agent, it should be used by a trained anaesthetist capable of dealing with an unconscious patient. The use of ketamine is limited by its side effects; sedation commonly lasts 6hr after its use and during this period most patients hallucinate. Post-traumatic stress syndrome is common in burns patients and many intermittently hallucinate with 'flashbacks' of the original trauma. Ketamine hallucinations superimposed on this can be very distressing.

### 9.4.1.5 *Oral opiates and haloperidol*

A neuroleptic technique involving the opiate fentanyl, given intravenously with the neuroleptic butyrophenone, droperidol, was used for many years to manage painful procedures such as burns dressings. This was successfully modified for several years to orally administered morphine and droperidol. Droperidol was withdrawn from the UK market, so the longer-acting neuroleptic haloperidol has been used instead. For this technique, the haloperidol is given 1–2hr before the dressing, whilst the morphine is given 30–60min before. In adults, a typical dose of 3–5mg haloperidol with 15–20mg morphine both given orally is used. Both these drugs are available as syrups and can be given through nasogastric and nasojejunal tubes. The key side effects of this regime are respiratory depression, sedation, and a 'locked in' sensation, where patients feel unable to move, although they are not in fact 'paralysed'. Despite this, the regime can be helpful and, compared to others, it has good patient acceptability.

Burns dressings continue to be a clinical problem, with no ideal regime that can be used with all patients. Sometimes, general anaesthesia is the only solution.

### 9.4.2 **Debridement and grafting**

Patients with major burns return to the operating theatre frequently to have debridment, removal of granulation and/or infected slough tissue, and then grafting. These procedures normally cause too much pain to be done without a general anaesthetic and cause significant post-operative pain. They also create periods of preoperative starvation and post-operative ileus that will interfere with both enteral feeding and oral medication. Local anaesthesia for these procedures would be helpful in minimizing all of these problems. Unfortunately, sepsis and heavy contamination of the skin with bacteria are contraindications to many of these techniques and so general anaesthesia is commonly preferred. Ketamine anaesthesia may also be used, although the prolonged sedation afterwards is unhelpful.

### 9.4.2.1 *The donor site*

Skin grafting causes severe post-operative pain at the donor site. This usually requires large doses of intravenous opiate for relief. Alternatively, the raw donor site may be covered with a gauze swab soaked in 0.25% bupivacaine with 1:200 000 adrenaline. This may then be covered with a waterproof layer, such as sterile paper or plastic, to stop evaporation and left for 10min before removal to apply the final dressing. The bupivacaine and adrenaline are adsorbed on to the raw and bleeding donor site, producing prolonged analgesia and vasoconstriction. Plasma bupivacaine levels have shown minimal systemic absorption over the first 6hr. This technique can provide complete pain relief for up to 8hr and dramatically reduce pain and opiate requirements.

## 9.5 **Central sensitization to pain**

Within the first 2 weeks after a major burn, patients commonly develop signs of central sensitization to pain, which usually persists until after all of the burn has been successfully skin grafted. The symptoms include

- Hyperpathia (increased intensity of pain from a painful stimulus)
- Allodynia (pain from stimuli which are not normally painful)
- Secondary hyperalgesia (increased pain sensitivity in surrounding undamaged tissue).

Even brushing the intact skin with bed linen causes excruciating pain.

Staff may misinterpret the symptoms of pain sensitization as 'attention-seeking', or 'a low pain threshold'. They need to be taught to recognize the symptoms, try to map out the areas affected and then handle these patients with great care, avoiding contact with the affected areas if possible.

Central pain sensitization may be mediated by the NMDA receptor, which is blocked by both dextromethorphan and ketamine. The use of low-dose ketamine infusions can reduce the incidence of pain sensitization significantly.

## 9.6 **Opiate tolerance**

Extensive burns will take several months of treatment to heal. Patients may be in severe pain for several weeks and need substantial doses of opiates to control their pain. Tolerance develops within the first few days and the daily dose of opiate needed for analgesia rises. Typically, when the daily dose of morphine exceeds 250mg, further increases have almost no effect. This situation may occur within 2 weeks of a major burn and creates a major problem for both patient and staff.

### 9.6.1 **Ultra-low-dose ketamine**

Based on animal experiments and a series of crossover experiments with PCA morphine and PCA ketamine, 'ultra-low-dose' ketamine infusions have been used to treat developed tolerance or to slow down its development in adults. As soon as major trauma or major burns patients are admitted to the hospital, morphine is initiated to treat their pain and 2mg/hr intravenous ketamine started at the same time. When used this way, the development of morphine tolerance is markedly slow and rarely becomes unmanageable.

Patients with unmanageable pain due to established opiate tolerance typically become more comfortable 6–8hr after starting the infusion. If the patient is pain-free, opiate doses will need to be reduced by 25% every 2 days until down to about 25% of the original dose, unless they are on PCA, when they will do their own dose reduction. If the ketamine is stopped whilst the patient is still in severe pain, opiate tolerance will develop again. On the other hand, if the patient's pain is mild to moderate, opiate consumption appears to stay constant.

Ketamine may alternatively be given orally in sweetened syrup at a dose of 25mg four times daily.

#### 9.6.1.1 *Side effects*

Even at this very low dose, there may be 'pressure of thought', visual disturbance, or sometimes hallucinations, although the latter may occur with post-traumatic stress syndrome as well. Anecdotally, patients seem to find these symptoms 'odd' rather than disturbing.

### 9.6.2 **Dependence**

Patients who have been on moderate to large doses of opiates for more than a week will develop a degree of physical dependence to their analgesics. If their analgesics are abruptly stopped, the patients develop a withdrawal syndrome, which may include flu-like symptoms, pallor, sweating, and abdominal pain. Patients may also become aggressive. These drugs should be tapered off over several days to avoid problems.

# References

Atchison NE, Osgood PF, Carr DB, and Szyfelbein SK (1991). Pain during burn dressing change in children: relationship to burn area, depth and analgesic regimens. *Pain*, **47**, 41–5.

Choiniere M, Grenier R, and Paquette C (1992). Patient-controlled analgesia: a double-blind study in burn patients. *Anaesthesia*, **47**, 467–72.

Coderre TJ and Melzack R (1987). Cutaneous hyperalgesia: contributions of the peripheral and central nervous system to the increase in pain sensitivity after injury. *Brain Research*, **404**, 95–106.

Collins HW, Jonsson CE, and Ericsson F (1995). Impairment of renal function after treatment of a burn patient with diclofenac, a non-steroidal anti-inflammatory drug. *Burns*, **21**, 471–3.

Davar G, Hama A, Deykin A, Vos B, and Maciewicz R (1991). MK-801 blocks the development of thermal hyperalgesia in a rat model of experimental painful neuropathy. *Brain Research*, **553**, 327–30.

Davies JW (1982). Prompt cooling of burned areas: a review of benefits and the effector mechanisms. *Burns Including Thermal Injury*, **9**, 1–6.

Demling RH, Ellerby S, and Jarrett F (1978). Ketamine analgesia for tangential excision of burn eschar: a burn unit procedure. *Journal of Trauma*, **18**, 269–70.

Donen N, Tweed WA, White D, Guttormson B, and Enns J (1982). Pre-hospital analgesia with entonox. *Canadian Anesthetists Society Journal*, **29**, 275–9.

Gaukroger PB, Chapman MJ, and Davey RB (1991). Pain control in paediatric burns—the use of patient-controlled analgesia. *Burns*, **17**, 396–9.

Gilboa D, Borenstein A, Seidman DS, and Tsur H (1990). Burn patients' use of autohypnosis: making a painful experience bearable. *Burns*, **16**, 441–4.

Groeneveld A and Inkson T (1992). Ketamine. A solution to procedural pain in burned children. *Canadian Nurse*, **88**, 28–31.

Ilkjaer S, Petersen KL, Brennum J, Wernberg M, and Dahl JB (1996). Effect of systemic N-methyl-D-aspartate receptor antagonist (ketamine) on primary and secondary hyperalgesia in humans. *British Journal of Anaesthesia*, **76**, 829–34.

McHugh GJ (1999). Norpethidine accumulation and generalized seizure during pethidine patient-controlled analgesia. *Anaesthesia and Intensive Care*, **27**, 289–91.

Patterson DR (1992). Practical applications of psychological techniques in controlling burn pain. *Journal of Burn Care & Rehabilitation*, **13**, 13–18.

Patterson DR, Questad KA, and de Lateur BJ (1989). Hypnotherapy as an adjunct to narcotic analgesia for the treatment of pain for burn debridement. *American Journal of Clinical Hypnosis*, **31**, 156–63.

Ptacek J, Patterson D, Montgomery B, and Heimbach D (1995). Pain, coping, and adjustment inpatients with burns: preliminary findings from a prospective study. *Journal of Pain and Symptom Management*, **10**, 446–55.

Quartaroli M, Fasdelli N, Bettelini L, Maraia G, and Corsi M (2001). GV196771A, an NMDA receptor/glycine site antagonist, attenuates mechanical allodynia in neuropathic rats and reduces tolerance induced by morphine in mice. *European Journal of Pharmacology*, **430**, 219–27.

Sinatra RS, Jahr JS, Reynolds LW, Viscusi ER, Groudine SB, and Payen-Champenois C (2005). Efficacy and safety of single and repeated administration of 1 gram intravenous acetaminophen injection (paracetamol) for pain management after major orthopedic surgery. *Anesthesiology*, **102**, 822–31.

Taal LA and Faber AW (1997). Post-traumatic stress, pain and anxiety in adult burn victims. *Burns*, **23**, 545–9.

# Chapter 10

# Acute pain in children

Richard F. Howard

### Key points

- Age and maturity affect the perception and expression of pain in children.
- A variety of pain assessment tools are needed to cover different age groups.
- The British National Formulary for Children is a source of correct formulations and doses of analgesics for children of different ages.
- Neonates show very high interindividual response to analgesic drugs.
- Between 2yrs and 12yrs, the clearance of drugs exceeds that of adults and relatively higher doses may be needed.
- Patient-controlled, nurse-controlled, and neuraxial analgesia can all be used in infants and children.
- Reducing procedural pain in children is important and requires a combination of pharmacological and non-pharmacological methods.

## 10.1 Introduction and general principles

To treat pain in children, it is important to understand how age and maturity influence the perception and expression of pain in children and how the effectiveness of analgesics and non-pharmacological management strategies differs at different ages.

The relief of pain in children should be a high priority for clinical staff who should receive appropriate and ongoing education and training in the assessment of pain and the elements of paediatric pain management. In many instances, acute pain is a predictable event, for example, after injury or surgery, and so protocols can be developed to standardize management and facilitate audit and control of the quality of care.

## 10.2 Assessment of pain

Good pain assessment is essential for effective pain management. Early recognition of pain can contribute to its prevention by prompting timely analgesia. A large number of measurement tools for use in children have been described; it is important to appreciate that no individual measure can be broadly recommended for pain assessment across all children or all contexts. A pain assessment tool must be valid for the age of the child, the setting in which it is to be used, and for the source and nature of pain.

There are three fundamental approaches to pain assessment in children: self-report, observational, and physiological.

*Self-report*: It is the only truly direct measure of pain; therefore, it is often considered the 'gold standard'. However, this method is not always reliable in children below the age of 4, as the ability to describe and quantify pain requires a level of understanding and communication that they may not possess. Self-report of pain is usually assisted by the use of a visual analogue scale (see Chapter 4). Older children and teenagers may be able to understand the concept of such scales and be able to use them successfully. Children younger than about 6yrs are unlikely to be able to do so, but they may benefit from the use of child friendly adaptations such as a graphical 'faces' type scale (see Figure 10.1).

*Observational/Behavioural*: Measuring behavioural distress associated with pain is a proxy measure of pain that must be used when self-report is impossible. A number of behaviours have been shown to be reliably associated with acute pain: a popular tool is the FLACC, as shown in Figure 10.1, valid for post-operative and procedural pain in children from ages 1yr to 18yrs.

*Physiological*: Measuring physiological arousal consequent to pain, such as heart rate, blood pressure, respiration, peripheral tissue oxygen saturation, plasma cortisol, or adrenaline, has been a popular approach, especially for neonates but it has very important limitations. Physiological measures alone should not be used to assess pain as they are very non-specific and liable to influence by homoeostatic mechanisms that will tend to reduce their responsiveness over time.

A full discussion of pain assessment for acute pain in children and advice on the selection of appropriate assessment tools for different clinical settings are available in guidelines published by the UK Royal College of Nursing Institute and the Association of Paediatric Anaesthetists of Great Britain and Ireland (RCN Institute, 1999; Howard R, Carter B, Curry J, et al, 2008).

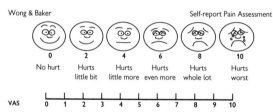

## Figure 10.1 Behavioral and self-report pain measurement tools

**FLACC**                          **Behavioural Pain Assessment**

| CATEGORIES | SCORING | | |
|---|---|---|---|
| | **0** | **1** | **2** |
| **Face** | No particular expression or smile | Occasional grimace or frown, withdrawn, disinterested | Frequent to constant quivering chin, clenched jaw |
| **Legs** | Normal position or relaxed | Uneasy, restless, tense | Kicking, or legs drawn up |
| **Activity** | Lying quietly, normal position, moves easily | Squirming, shifting back and forth, tense | Arched, rigid or jerking |
| **Cry** | No cry (awake or asleep) | Moans or whimpers, occasional complaint | Crying steadily, screams or sobs, frequent complaints |
| **Consolability** | Content, relaxed | Reassured by occasional touching, hugging or being talked to, distractible | Difficult to console or comfort |

Each of the five categories: **(F)** Face; **(L)** Legs; **(A)** Activity; **(C)** Cry; **(C)** Consolability; is scored from 0–2 which results in a total score between 0 and 10

**Wong & Baker**                       **Self-report Pain Assessment**

| 0 | 2 | 4 | 6 | 8 | 10 |
|---|---|---|---|---|---|
| No hurt | Hurts little bit | Hurts little more | Hurts even more | Hurts whole lot | Hurts worst |

**VAS**    0   1   2   3   4   5   6   7   8   9   10

Adapted from Wong DL, Baker CM (1988). Pain in children: comparison of assessment scales. *Okla Nursing*, **33**, 8; and Merkel SI, Voepel-Lewis T, Shayevitz JR, Malviya S (1997). The FLACC: a behavioral scale for scoring postoperative pain in young children. *Pediatric Nursing*, **23**, 293–27.

## 10.3 Analgesics and analgesic techniques

Analgesic regimens should normally incorporate combinations of analgesics and non-pharmacological methods of pain management that are appropriate to the perceived or expected level of pain. Frequent pain assessments to evaluate pain and the response to analgesia are essential, they should be documented to demonstrate the effectiveness of treatments and guide ongoing therapy. Analgesia must be sufficiently potent and flexible to allow for interindividual differences in response and variations in the intensity of pain that can occur depending on the circumstances. Correct analgesic dosages and drug formulations suitable for children of different ages should be verified by consulting specialist paediatric resources such as the BNFC (The British National Formulary for Children 2009), many of which are available online.

### 10.3.1 **Developmental pharmacology**

Body composition changes markedly with age, which has implications for both the volume of distribution (VD) of analgesics and their clearance (CL). Total body water is 85% of body weight at 32 weeks gestation, close to 80% at 35 weeks, and 75% at birth, falling to 70% in the first post-natal week, and then more slowly to about 50–60%, similar to adult values, by 18 months. Extracellular water steadily declines from 40% of body weight to 25% by puberty. Body fat is about 12% body weight in the term neonate, increasing to 25% by 1yr and then falling to about 15% at 7–8yrs. Thereafter, there is a slow but sustained increase in body fat that is greater in girls and reaches a plateau in the non-obese adult. Plasma proteins, albumin, and $\alpha_1$-acid glycoprotein are reduced in the neonate increasing VD for some drugs; higher levels of unbound drugs are also more likely to cause toxic effects particularly after rapid intravenous injection (e.g. after accidental intravascular injection of local anaesthetics). Hepatic enzyme function is also developmentally regulated such that biotransformation reactions and conjugation may be reduced or incomplete, particularly in the first months of life. Renal function is also reduced at birth; glomerular filtration rates are approximately 10% of adult values at term, and renal tubular secretion does not reach mature values until 6 months of age, contributing to the reduced clearance and prolonged elimination half-life ($t_{1/2}$) seen for renally excreted drugs.

### 10.3.2 **Analgesic dosing in the neonate and infant**

Pharmacokinetic variables are important determinants of suitable doses and dosage regimens. In addition, the neonatal period is characterized by very high interindividual variability such that the efficacy and side effects of many drugs can be unpredictable.

In general, CL for analgesics is relatively low in neonates and so maintenance doses (mg/kg) must be reduced, and dosage intervals increased to prevent accumulation. Clearance increases in infancy, reaching or exceeding adult levels by 6 months to 1yr. Between 2yrs and 12yrs, CL is high compared with older children and adults; therefore, maintenance doses and infusion rates may need to be increased to maintain adequate plasma levels.

#### 10.3.2.1 *Paracetamol*

Paracetamol is probably the most widely used analgesic for children of all ages. It is safe and effective for mild pain and useful in combination with other analgesics when pain is more severe. Paracetamol is available as an oral suspension, tablets, capsules, rectal suppository, and intravenous solution. The pharmacology of paracetamol has been relatively well investigated, the required dose depends on both age and route of administration but should not exceed 90mg/kg/day, and less in neonates (see Table 10.1). Dose-related hepatotoxicity is the most serious adverse effect of paracetamol; it has mostly been reported with single doses greater than 150mg/kg, but as accumulation can occur it is not recommended that paracetamol be continued for more than 5 days at maximum doses without close medical supervision.

| Table 10.1 Analgesics for mild to moderate pain | | | |
|---|---|---|---|
| Drug | Class of analgesic | Route of administration | Doses |
| Paracetamol | Antipyretic–analgesic | Oral/rectal | 15–20mg/kg qid 90mg/kg/day max. (60mg/kg/day term neonate) (30–45mg/kg/day pre-term) |
| | | Intravenous | 10–15mg/kg qid 40mg/kg/day term neonate 60mg/kg/day < 50kg body weight 4g daily > 50kg |
| Ibuprofen | NSAID | Oral | 20mg/kg/day <6 months 30mg/kg/day >6 months (max. 2.4g/day) |
| Diclofenac | NSAID | Oral | 1mg/kg tid (3mg/kg/day) |
| | | Rectal | 1mg/kg tid (3mg/kg/day) |
| Ketorolac | NSAID | Oral | 0.5–1mg/kg qid (max. 10mg/dose) Max daily dose 150mg |
| | | Intravenous | 0.5mg/kg qid (max. 10mg/dose) Max daily dose 150mg |
| Codeine | Opioid | Oral | 1mg/kg qid |
| | | Rectal | 1mg/kg qid Max daily dose 240mg |
| | | Intravenous | Not recommended |
| Tramadol | Opioid/monoaminergic | Oral | 1–2mg/kg qid |
| | | Intravenous | 1mg/kg qid Max daily dose 600mg |

### 10.3.2.2 *NSAIDs*

Ibuprofen, diclofenac, and ketorolac have been used extensively for acute pain in children, although ketorolac is not popular in some countries because it is perceived as more likely to be associated with adverse effects such as bleeding or renal impairment. Ibuprofen is probably the safest, it is certainly the best investigated (see Table 10.1 for doses). Non-steroidal anti-inflammatory drugs (NSAIDs) are known to have a number of important side effects that can influence their indications. Acute renal failure, especially in the very dehydrated or young, can occur after relative overdose. Changes in platelet function can cause increased bleeding tendency, and cross-sensitivity with aspirin-induced asthma is possible. Renal toxicity can generally be avoided by observing recommended doses and maintaining fluid balance. The use of NSAIDs is controversial after some kinds of surgery where bleeding is a particular problem, notably tonsillectomy. Ibuprofen appears to be a relatively safer choice, and more recent analyses of clinical studies appear to indicate that judicious use of ibuprofen after tonsillectomy is safe and does not increase the rate of re-operation for bleeding. Aspirin-induced asthma is much more rare in children than adults, but as aspirin is not generally given to children (because it can cause Reye's syndrome), families of children with asthma are not usually aware of the presence or absence of aspirin sensitivity. However, large population studies of children including those with asthma and respiratory tract infections have again demonstrated that ibuprofen is very safe. Some authorities recommend that NSAIDs should not be used during acute exacerbations of asthma unless the patient is definitely known not to be sensitive. NSAIDs are not usually prescribed for pain in infants less than 3 months old, although they have been used for closure of patent ductus arteriosus in premature neonates where the benefit–risk is felt to be more acceptable.

### 10.3.2.3 *Opioids: NCA and PCA*

Opioids are used at all ages for moderate and severe pain. Moderate potency opioids such as codeine and tramadol are popular by the oral route, where they are given in combination with paracetamol and NSAIDs (Table 10.1). The efficacy of codeine is rather unpredictable, particularly if given as a sole analgesic, as it is a prodrug that normally undergoes metabolism to morphine. As many as 40% of children may not have normal metabolizing capacity, and up to 10% may be incapable of converting codeine to morphine. It should, therefore, only be used where its effects can be confidently assessed.

Although the oral route is generally preferred when available, higher potency opioids can be used by a variety of routes (Table 10.2). Parenteral opioid infusions are frequently used for moderate to severe pain, for example, after surgery (Tables 10.3 and 10.4). Such

| Table 10.2 Initial doses for potent opioids | | |
|---|---|---|
| Morphine | Oral | 0.1mg/kg (<1 month) |
| | | 0.2mg/kg (>1 month) |
| | | Max initial dose 20mg |
| | Intravenous | 20–50mcg/kg (<1 month) |
| | | 50–100mcg/kg (>1 month) |
| | Subcutaneous | 0.05mg/kg |
| | Epidural | 20–50mcg/kg |
| Oxycodone | Oral | 0.2mg/kg |
| Hydrocodone | Oral | 0.2mg/kg |
| Methadone | Oral | 0.2mg/kg |
| | Intravenous | 0.1–0.2mg/kg |

| Table 10.3 Morphine infusion for neonates (age <1 month) | |
|---|---|
| Preparation | Morphine sulphate 1mg/kg in 50mL solution |
| Concentration | 20mcg/kg/mL (0.02mg/kg/mL) |
| Initial dose | 0.5–2.5mL (10–50mcg/kg) |
| Infusion rate | 0.1–0.6mL/hr (2–12mcg/kg/hr) |

| Table 10.4 Morphine infusion (age >1 month) | |
|---|---|
| Preparation | Morphine sulphate 1mg/kg in 50mL solution |
| Concentration | 20mcg/kg/mL (0.02mg/kg/mL) |
| Initial dose | 1.0–5.0mL (20–100mcg/kg) |
| Infusion rate | 0.5–1.5mL/hr (10–30mcg/kg/hr) |

infusions are safe provided adequate systems of supervision and monitoring are in place. Nurse-controlled analgesia (NCA) is an infusion system using patient-controlled analgesia (PCA) technology that will allow extra doses of analgesia to be given at the discretion of the bedside nurse; suitable regimens are given in Table 10.5. PCA can be used for children older than 6yrs of age provided they are willing to use the handset, and are capable of understanding the concept. Children using PCA need relatively closer monitoring and more regular reminders of when to use the handset compared to adults. It is common to use a small continuous 'background' infusion throughout as this is thought to improve the overall quality of analgesia without unduly compromising safety (Table 10.6).

| Table 10.5 **NCA** | |
|---|---|
| **Preparation** | Morphine sulphate 1mg/kg in 50mL solution |
| Concentration | 20mcg/kg/mL |
| Initial dose | 2.5–5.0 mL (50–100mcg/kg) |
| *Programming* | |
| Background infusion | 0.5–1.0mL/hr (10–20mcg/kg/hr) |
| NCA dose | 0.5–1.0mL (10–20mcg/kg) |

| Table 10.6 **PCA** | |
|---|---|
| **Preparation** | Morphine sulphate 1mg/kg in 50mL solution |
| Concentration | 20mcg/kg/mL |
| Initial dose | 2.5–5.0mL (50–100mg/kg) |
| *Programming* | |
| Background infusion | 0–0.2mL/hr (0–4mcg/kg/hr) |
| PCA dose | 0.5–1.0mL (10–20mcg/kg/hr) |

### 10.3.3 **Local anaesthesia**

Local anaesthesia (LA) plays an extremely important role in paediatric acute pain management from topical anaesthesia of the skin for venepuncture and minor procedures, to peripheral and central nerve blocks for surgery and post-operative analgesia. Even simple post-operative infiltration of the surgical wound can reduce requirements for further analgesia after laparoscopic surgery and after relatively minor procedures such as inguinal hernia repair or dental extractions. Levobupivacaine and in some circumstances ropivacaine have largely replaced bupivacaine as the preferred local anaesthetic due to their slightly improved safety profile. When used in equivalent concentrations levobupivacaine is almost indistinguishable from bupivacaine in clinical practice.

#### 10.3.3.1 *Simple nerve blocks*

Penile dorsal nerve block, ilioinguinal/iliohypogastric block, and caudal epidural block are the most useful LA procedures because so much routine surgery in children is confined to the region below the umbilicus. Detailed technical descriptions are available in standard texts (Peutrell and Mather 1997; Howard 2002); the blocks are easy to learn and very safe. Ultrasound guidance may further improve their accuracy, safety, and success rates. The principal drawback of these blocks is their limited duration, although they do cover the short period during post-operative recovery when oral medication is not possible.

### 10.3.3.2 *Neuraxial analgesics*

In recent years, there has been considerable interest in prolonging the duration of caudal block by adding neuraxially effective analgesics such as ketamine or clonidine to the LA. There is no doubt that both of these compounds are capable of prolonging the duration of analgesia after a single caudal dose for 8–24hr. Commonly recommended doses are clonidine 1–2mcg/kg (1mcg/kg or less in neonates), or ketamine 0.5mg/kg. Unfortunately, as neither of these compounds is licensed for neuraxial use in children, neither has undergone the rigorous safety testing for potential neurotoxicity that this would require; and so there has been ongoing debate about the prudence of routine administration. Nevertheless, both have been in fairly common use in some parts of the world for quite some time and few problems have been reported. Higher doses can lead to dangerous or unpleasant side effects including excessive sedation and hypotension for clonidine, and adverse neuro-behavioural effects for ketamine.

### 10.3.3.3 *Complex and continuous nerve blocks*

More complex blocks such as brachial plexus, paravertebral, lumbar, or thoracic epidurals are indicated for specialist surgery; and when extensive prolonged and intense analgesia is required catheters are usually left in place so that analgesia can be infused. These blocks are more complicated to perform and more prone to difficulties and complications. Continuous blocks, although very effective, can only be unreservedly recommended when fully trained support is continuously available. Technical details can be found elsewhere (Peutrell and Mather 1997).

### 10.3.3.4 *Continuous epidural analgesia*

Lumbar and thoracic epidural analgesia is indicated for major surgery of the thorax, abdomen spine, and lower limbs. Epidurals in children are always sited under general anaesthesia. In children weighing 10kg or greater, an 18g normal, adult, 10cm long Tuohy needle is suitable, and for smaller children and infants, a shorter 5cm long needle is available. Both of these will accept a 21g catheter; finer catheters that are subject to more technical problems, such as sudden blockage or kinking, are not recommended. Catheters can also be threaded to higher, even thoracic, segments from the technically easier to access caudal space but for all sites of access (caudal, lumbar, or thoracic) if the catheter is advanced more than a few centimetres then it is advisable to confirm its position. The location of the catheter tip can be found using a number of methods including X-ray imaging with radio-opaque contrast, electrostimulation, ultrasound, or ECG measurement. Special catheters or equipment may be required.

For post-operative analgesia, LA with or without opioid is commonly infused depending somewhat on the clinical setting and local preferences. Overall, there is slightly stronger evidence to support the use of hydrophilic opioid, such as morphine or hydromorphone, in comparison with lipophilic opioids such as fentanyl (Howard *et al.* 2008); however, satisfactory conditions can be achieved with either (Table 10.7).

As with all complex blocks, patients must be nursed in a safe and suitable environment and cared for by trained staff who are competent in the assessment and management of epidural analgesia. Because epidural opioids can have prolonged or delayed effects, it is usual to continue specialist care and monitoring for 12–24hr after the infusion is discontinued. The potential complications are daunting and may include LA toxicity, cardiorespiratory collapse, epidural infection, excessive motor block, stasis-related skin breakdown, and others; all of which can be avoided with good care.

## 10.4 Management of painful procedures

Routine medical care involving intravenous access, blood sampling, and other painful diagnostic and therapeutic procedures can cause great distress for children and their families. When such procedures are essential, it is important that they should be achieved with as little pain as possible. General considerations when planning procedural pain management are as follows:

- Are sedation or even general anaesthesia likely to be required for a safe and satisfactory outcome?
- Would modification of the procedure reduce pain? For example, venepuncture is less painful than heel lance for infant blood sampling

| Table 10.7 Epidural infusion regimens | |
|---|---|
| **(1) Levobupivacaine–morphine** | |
| Initial dose | Levobupivacaine 0.25%:0.5–0.75mL/kg |
| Infusion | Levobupivacaine 0.125% with preservative-free morphine 0.001% |
| Rate | 0.1–0.4mL/hr* |
| **(2) Levobupivacaine–fentanyl** | |
| Initial dose | Levobupivacaine 0.25%:0.5–0.75mL/kg |
| Infusion | Levobupivacaine 0.125% with fentanyl 1–2mcg/mL |
| Rate | 0.1–0.4mL/hr* |
| **(3) Ropivacaine** | |
| Initial dose | Ropivacaine 0.2%:0.5–0.75mL/kg |
| Infusion | Ropivacaine 0.2% |
| Rate | 0.1–0.4mL/hr* |
| * Maximum rate 0.2mL/hr in neonates. | |

- Is the planned environment suitable? Ideally this should be a quiet, calm place with suitable toys and distractions
- Allow sufficient time for analgesic drugs and other analgesic measures to be effective
- Ensure that appropriate personnel are available, and enlist experienced help when necessary
- Formulate a clear plan of action should the procedure fail or pain become unmanageable using the techniques selected
- Procedural pain management should generally include a combination of pharmacological and non-pharmacological approaches to pain management using developmentally appropriate techniques. Distraction, hypnosis, and guided imagery are examples of behavioural techniques that have been shown to be effective for brief pain. Sucrose reduces pain responses in neonates and is safe and simple to administer. These measures can be combined with topical local anaesthesia or systemic analgesia as appropriate. Detailed descriptions of the management of a number of different procedures are given in 'Good Practice in Postoperative and Procedural Pain', a guideline recently published by the Association of Paediatric Anaesthetists of Great Britain and Ireland.

# References

Howard RF (2002). Practical applications and procedures. In Breivik H, Campbell W, and Eccleston C, eds. *Procedures for Pediatric Pain Management*, pp. 431–45. Arnold, London.

Howard R, Carter B, Curry J, et al. (2008). Good Practice in Postoperative and Procedural Pain Management. *Pediatric Anesthesia*, **18**, 1–78.

Peutrell JM and Mather SJ (1997). *Regional Anaesthesia in Babies and Children*. Oxford University Press, Oxford, UK.

Royal College of Nursing Institute. (1999). *The Recognition and Assessment of Pain in Children*. Royal college of Nursing, London. Available at www.rcn.org.uk/development/practice/clinicalguidelines/pain (last accessed).

The British National Formulary for Children. (2009). BMJ Publishing Group Ltd., London. Available at http://bnfc.org/bnfc/

# Chapter 11

# Acute pain in the elderly

Adrian Wagg and Shashi Gadgil

## Key points

- Physiological changes that occur with age affect the pharmacokinetics and pharmacodynamics of drugs used in acute pain management.
- Elderly patients are often reluctant to complain of pain and seek treatment and may sometimes be unable to express pain due to impaired cognition or language.
- Evidence suggests the elderly as a group that receive inadequate analgesia and are often in pain.
- Health care professionals are often reluctant to administer sufficient analgesia due to fear of encouraging addiction or inducing side effects.
- The approach to pain management in this group should follow the World Health Organization (WHO) analgesic ladder with close monitoring for potential side effects and with escalation of treatment till sufficient analgesia is achieved.
- Choice of drugs and the route of administration should be tailored to the individual patient and should consider the nature of their pain and any disability or co-morbidity that will affect their response to the chosen agent.
- Non-steroidal anti-inflammatory drugs (NSAIDs) should be used with extreme caution, monitoring for potential gastrointestinal (GI) and renal side effects and long-term use should be avoided if possible.
- Opioids are effective analgesics and should not be denied to the elderly but their use should be monitored carefully and side effects such as nausea and constipation anticipated and treated.

# 11.1 Physiological changes in the elderly

## 11.1.1 Cardiovascular

Fifty to sixty-five per cent of elderly patients have cardiovascular disease, although in some patients the disease may be completely asymptomatic. Cardiac output declines by about 1% per year over the age of 30 and small changes in intravascular volume or venous capacitance may induce cardiovascular instability. Hypovolaemia or the reduced sympathetic response following epidural anaesthesia can induce a profound reduction in cardiac output in the elderly; this reduced cardiac output leads to reduced hepatic and renal blood flow which in turn affects drug clearance. It also leads to higher peak arterial concentrations of intravenously administered drugs such as morphine.

## 11.1.2 Renal

Glomerular filtration rate (GFR) decreases by 1–1.5% per year after the age of 20. Total renal blood flow decreases by 10% per decade. Tubular excretion and reabsorption, renal metabolism, and clearance of drugs and metabolites are affected by ageing. Measurements of serum creatinine levels are an unreliable assessment of GFR due to reduced muscle mass with ageing. Creatinine clearance is the most reliable indicator of GFR. Estimated GFRs produced automatically from routine biochemistry are a useful guide to renal function in older people but caution should be exercised in the very elderly or malnourished.

## 11.1.3 Hepatic and digestive function

Routine liver function tests remain steady in old age despite the fact that liver perfusion falls by about 40% and liver size by approximately 30% and drug metabolism can be affected. Gastrointestinal (GI) physiological function is usually maintained. Gastric prostaglandin synthesis, bicarbonate and non-parietal fluid secretion may diminish and *Helicobacter pylori* infestation is common. These factors make the elderly more susceptible to non-steroidal anti-inflammatory drug (NSAID)-induced mucosal damage.

## 11.1.4 Peripheral and central nervous system

Neuronal and neurotransmitter activity and density within the cholinergic and dopaminergic systems and the number of neurotransmitter receptor sites in nerve tissue decreases with age. A decrease in the rate of synthesis of neurotransmitters and fibrosis of neurons in sympathoadrenal pathways causes a decline in sympathetic response. Despite this, plasma levels of catecholamines are actually higher in the elderly patient although this may not be clinically apparent due to the age-related decrease in autonomic responsiveness. Self-regulation of the autonomic nervous system is impaired so that techniques which cause rapid loss of sympathetic activity, such as spinal and epidural anaesthesia, are more likely to produce significant hypotension in elderly patients than in young patients.

There is an age-dependent reduction in β-endorphin content and gamma-aminobutyric acid (GABA) synthesis in the lateral thalamus and a decline in the concentration of GABA and serotonin receptors. C and Aδ pain fibre function deteriorates with age causing a decrease in the speed and capacity of processing of painful stimuli. Loss or atrophy of peripheral nerves also causes slowing of nerve conduction in motor fibres.

## 11.2 Pharmacodynamic and pharmacokinetic changes in the elderly

### 11.2.1 Absorption

Slowed intestinal transit time in the elderly increases available time for drug absorption; however, this is offset by reduced jejunal surface area and blood flow to the GI tract. Transdermal routes appear to be equally efficient in the elderly as in younger patients despite changes in skin composition associated with ageing. Transbuccal absorption may decrease if saliva output falls. Transbronchial absorption appears to be similar in all ages. Response to local anaesthetics is affected by the neural changes mentioned above. Intramuscular administration is best avoided in the elderly as absorption is unpredictable due to change in fat/muscle ratio.

### 11.2.2 Distribution

The distribution of drugs in the elderly is affected by reduced muscle mass and body water and increased fat mass. Fat acts as a depot for lipophilic drugs such as fentanyl and lidocaine, thus prolonging their duration of action. Water-soluble drugs such as morphine sulphate are less efficiently distributed and higher plasma concentrations are obtained with equivalent doses; thus, side effects such as oversedation and respiratory depression are more common. Decreases in serum albumin due to chronic disease and malnutrition increase free drug availability. This increases the potential for adverse effects with highly protein-bound analgesics such as NSAIDs and anti-epileptic agents.

### 11.2.3 Drug elimination

The physiological changes to the liver and kidneys discussed earlier mean that elderly patients are less effective at clearing drugs from the bloodstream. Drugs that undergo extensive first pass metabolism, such as lidocaine and opiates, may exhibit a rise in peak plasma concentrations.

Hepatic phase 1 reactions involving oxidation, hydrolysis, and reduction appear more strongly altered by age than phase 2 conjugation processes. In general, phase 1 reactions diminish irrespective of which microsomal cytochrome P450 enzyme is involved, although there is variation between individual drugs. Paracetamol and diazepam, both processed through the same enzymatic routes, are metabolized at equal rates regardless of age. Carbamazepine, lidocaine, and fentanyl are subject to reduced metabolism by the same enzyme systems in older adults. Age appears to have no effect on the frequencies of slow and rapid-metabolizing genetic polymorphisms.

Reduction in renal clearance is the most important pharmacodynamic effect of ageing. Even if baseline renal function is normal, illness, dehydration, and the use of nephrotoxic drugs will cause renal impairment and affect drug clearance.

### 11.2.4 **Pharmacodynamic changes**

The number of receptors present in tissues and/or the affinity of these receptors for neurotransmitters decrease with age. Elderly patients are therefore more susceptible to the effects of opioids and benzodiazepines. The prescription of antipsychotics and some antiemetics may induce extrapyramidal reactions due to the reduction in central dopaminergic neurons, receptor numbers, and dopamine concentrations. Anticholinergic side effects are also more readily seen because muscarinic receptor numbers and acetylcholine levels fall with age. Animal experiments also suggest that μ- and κ-opioid receptor numbers fall while δ-opioid receptor numbers are unchanged. Impairment of physiological and homoeostatic mechanisms, including autonomic dysfunction, impaired thermoregulation, and reduced cognitive function, put the elderly at risk of symptomatic orthostatic reactions, falls, and confusion after the administration of potentially sedating drugs. There may be synergistic effects if more than one class of drug is used.

## 11.3 **Special considerations in the elderly**

### 11.3.1 **Assessment and reporting of pain**

Many elderly people believe that pain is a part of growing old and accept that this is the case. This may influence the way they report pain, seek help, and comply with the treatment. The elderly are also often reluctant to acknowledge and address the contribution of psychological factors that influence such pain behaviour.

### 11.3.2 **Dementia and acute confusional states**

Cognitive impairment reduces the patient's ability to express and localize acute pain and to seek relief. Research that has focused on pain in those with cognitive impairment has consistently shown that this group under-reports pain when compared with their peers who have no cognitive impairment and that those with better cognitive functioning are more likely to receive analgesics than others. In addition to enduring physical pain needlessly, patients with dementia can express challenging behaviour that is directly related to the lack of pain management. The more confused and disorientated the patient with dementia is, the fewer analgesics they are likely to be prescribed and administered. Screaming, verbal and physical aggression, agitation, and wandering by patients present significant challenges to staff providing care in acute hospital settings. This behaviour is often associated with the presence of pain in those with dementia. Frequently, the primary response to this is treatment with an antipsychotic medication. This can mask symptoms that are related to pain, prevent effective treatment, and may affect recovery time. Prescription of pain relief does not necessarily mean that analgesics are administered, as even when pain relief medication is prescribed to patients with dementia, up to 83% do not receive it. This may be attributed to a combination of a lack of education in this area amongst health care professionals, fear of side effects, fear of causing addiction, and doubting the reliability of patients with dementia to accurately report pain.

Older, cognitively impaired patients have been shown reliably and validly to rate their pain, so asking the patient should always be the first step in assessment. In those with verbal communication difficulties, there are a number of pain assessment tools and scoring systems that can be used such as the Abbey pain scale (Abbey et al. 2004 or the Assessment of Discomfort in Dementia Protocol (Kovach et al. 1999 These assess and score the likelihood that the patient is in pain by looking at facial expression, verbalization, body movement, changes in interpersonal interaction, changes in activity patterns, or routines and changes in mental status (Table 11.1). It is also important to ask relatives and carers about any particular patterns of behaviour associated with pain in individual cases. The familiar undergraduate teaching about rating the amount of pain on a scale from 1 to 10 is unreliable in a significant proportion of older people.

Once pain has been identified in this group, regular drug treatment should be prescribed according to the analgesic ladder. The response to this can be assessed and treatment reviewed regularly. As required regimes should be avoided for the reasons outlined above. Other factors such as nursing in a calm and unstressful environment and good positioning should also be considered.

## 11.4 **Analgesic drugs in the elderly**

The pharmacology of these drugs has been discussed in earlier chapters so this section will focus on issues specific to the elderly.

| Table 11.1 Areas of observation for pain assessment | |
|---|---|
| **Physiological observation** | |
| • Change in colour | • Change in pulse rate |
| • Change in blood pressure | • Change in temperature |
| • Loss of appetite or fluid intake | • Change in respiratory rate |
| • Urinary or faecal incontinence | • Change in sleeping pattern |
| • Sweating | • Guarding the painful area |
| **Behavioural observation** | |
| • Aggression | • Increased movement |
| • Agitation | • Decreased movement |
| • Reaction to touch | • Not weight bearing |
| • Weeping or moaning | • Increased confusion |
| • Shouting | • Unable to settle |
| **Body language** | |
| • Facial expression | • Withdrawal |
| • Assume foetal position | • Knee(s) drawn up |

Source: Cunningham C (2006). Managing pain in patients with dementia in hospital. *Nursing Standard*, 20, 54–8.

### 11.4.1 Paracetamol

Paracetamol (acetaminophen) is used as an analgesic and antipyretic. There is no dose alteration required for elderly patients. The American College of Rheumatologists guidelines recommend it as first-line therapy due to its low cost, broad tolerability, reasonable efficacy, and a low side-effect profile. It has very few drug interactions, an important consideration due to polypharmacy in this age group. It should be used with caution in patients with known liver disease; however, there is no absolute contraindication to a short course of paracetamol under medical supervision in this group.

### 11.4.2 NSAIDs and COX-2 inhibitors

NSAIDs and selective inhibitors of cyclooxygenase 2 have useful analgesic and antipyretic effects at low doses that are seen soon after administration. Their anti-inflammatory effects are seen at higher doses and with sustained use. NSAIDs should be used with caution in the elderly due to their wide range of adverse effects.

GI effects are due to the inhibition of prostaglandin synthesis by cyclooxygenase inhibition. Prostaglandins are important in maintaining GI mucosal integrity and reduced production leads to inflammation, ulceration, or even perforation of gastric mucosa. A significant number of people suffer fatal GI haemorrhage each year as a consequence and this often occurs without warning symptoms of abdominal pain or dyspepsia. The elderly are at higher risk due to lower baseline levels of prostaglandin synthesis. Concomitant use of aspirin and anticoagulants for cardiovascular disease further increases the risk. Concomitant prescription of gastroprotective agents such as prostaglandin analogues, proton pump inhibitors, or $H_2$ receptor antagonists can reduce the risk of GI side effects but they may also mask warning signs of GI side effects; in one study of long-term NSAID use in elderly patients, those on $H_2$ antagonists had 2.5 times more hospitalizations with GI complications than those on no GI protective agents. COX-2 inhibitors should, in theory, have fewer side effects but similar adverse effects to the NSAIDs can occur.

Renal effects of NSAIDs are also due to prostaglandin inhibition. Prostaglandins are important in the maintenance of renal blood flow during times of volume depletion. In patients with heart failure, renal impairment, hepatic dysfunction, or intravascular volume depletion, the administration of NSAIDs may therefore precipitate acute renal failure. Renal prostaglandins also have an important role in regulating sodium reabsorption in the loop of Henle. Inhibition of these prostaglandins may result in increased sodium reabsorption, which then causes fluid retention. This could manifest as peripheral oedema or it may cause a clinical deterioration in patients with pre-existing heart failure, renal impairment, or hypertension. NSAIDs may also decrease the efficacy of β-blockers, ACE inhibitors, and diuretics. The incidence of adverse renal and cardiovascular events remains significant with the COX-2 inhibitors.

Platelet dysfunction is a common effect of NSAIDs, and as in the case of aspirin for vascular ischaemic events is often desirable. Aspirin irreversibly inhibits platelets so the effect lasts the lifespan of the platelet, usually 7–14 days. Most NSAIDs also cause platelet dysfunction, but this is reversible and platelet function returns after the drugs are discontinued. COX-2 inhibitors do not affect platelet aggregation in doses used in clinical practice. In elderly patients on oral anticoagulant therapy, NSAIDs should be used with extreme caution and avoided where possible.

Other effects of NSAIDs that are less commonly appreciated include central nervous system disturbance, such as sedation, confusion, cognitive dysfunction, psychosis, and personality changes. These reverse when the drug is stopped. Dizziness and tinnitus have also been described.

The pharmacology of the various NSAIDs is discussed in Chapter 2. Those commonly used in the United Kingdom include aspirin, ibuprofen, naproxen, ketorolac, indometacin, diclofenac, and piroxicam. These are mostly oral preparations except for ketorolac and some preparations of diclofenac which can be given by intravenous bolus injection. Diclofenac can be given intramuscularly and *per rectum*. Celecoxib and etoricoxib are the COX-2 inhibitors licensed for use in the United Kingdom.

Choice of agent is mostly dependent on cost, duration of action, and route of administration. In the elderly, it is advisable to use the lowest dose for the shortest possible time, monitoring closely for adverse effects. Dose reduction is required in patients with liver disease as most NSAIDs are metabolized by the liver.

### 11.4.3 Opioids

Strong opioids are efficacious in acute severe pain such as that occurring after surgery. The weaker opioids tend to be used for chronic pain syndromes. A substantial body of evidence in addition to everyday practical experience informs us that opioids provide useful pain relief in a broad range of conditions. A major influence on the decision to use these drugs in the elderly is the risk of side effects.

*Nausea and vomiting* occur in 25% of patients after the administration of strong opioids. A prophylactic anti-emetic should always be administered simultaneously to avoid problems with patient compliance. If strong opioids are used on a chronic basis, anti-emetics may only need to be given for the first 5 days of treatment. It is logical to give longer-acting anti-emetics such as ondansetron if long acting opioids are used.

*Constipation* is almost inevitable with long-term opioid use and prophylaxis with faecal softeners and stimulant laxatives should be given.

*Pruritus* is most common after intrathecal and epidural administration but may complicate oral and parenteral use. It usually responds to antihistamines such as chlorpheniramine.

*Tolerance* is common with opioids but can be avoided if these drugs are only used for short periods. Adjuvant drugs can be used to minimize the amount of opioid required or the different types of opioid drugs can be rotated. As tolerance occurs, the dose needs to be increased to achieve the same analgesic effect, often there is also increased tolerance to the principal side effects of the drug.

#### 11.4.3.1 Cognitive and motor function

Effects are most marked in the early stages of opioid treatment. A single dose of morphine has been shown to significantly reduce motor task reaction time. Other adverse effects include mental clouding, sedation, and confusion, which may be acceptable for the short term in the acute hospital setting. In the longer term, stable use of sustained release morphine and transdermal fentanyl is not associated with impairment of cognitive or motor performance. However, these functions may be temporarily impaired when opioids are initiated and also when doses are increased. If elderly patients do require strong opioids, then aiming to achieve a steady serum level of drug with controlled release preparations is the best way to minimize these effects.

*Respiratory depression* is a side effect seen in overdose, this can be avoided by cautious upward dose titration. The pharmacology of the various opioids is discussed in Chapter 2. Weak opioids commonly used in the United Kingdom include codeine, dihydrocodeine, dextropropoxyphene, and tramadol. Stronger opioids include morphine, diamorphine, hydromorphone, methadone, buprenorphine, and oxycodone.

### 11.4.4 Tricyclic antidepressants

There is a high incidence of depression in older people and in people with chronic pain. There is considerable evidence that tricyclic antidepressants (TCAs) also have analgesic effects independent of the effect on mood. Their use is well established in the treatment of pain due to diabetic neuropathy, postherpetic neuralgia, trigeminal neuralgia, tension headache, migraine, fibromyalgia, and low back pain. Amitriptyline, imipramine, doxepin, clomipramine, desipramine, and nortriptyline have all been extensively studied. They do have a wide range of adverse effects and drug interactions that are particularly problematical in the elderly. Most are sedating, cause anticholinergic side effects such as dry mouth and constipation, and can cause marked postural hypotension. They are contraindicated in patients with significant cardiac arrhythmias, bladder outflow tract obstruction, prostatic hypertrophy, and narrow-angle glaucoma. Extreme caution is advised in using TCAs in this patient group. If they are to be used, the minimum dose should be initiated, usually at bedtime with a slow dose titration watching for side effects.

### 11.4.5 Anti-epileptic drugs

Some of the drugs used commonly in epilepsy have also been shown to be beneficial in treating neuropathic pain. The most commonly used are carbamazepine and gabapentin. Side effects seen in the elderly include cognitive impairment and sedation with all the anti-epileptics and fluid retention and hyponatraemia with carbamazepine.

### 11.4.6 Muscle relaxants

These can be used to improve spasticity, reduce muscle spasm, or treat pain. Spasticity from upper motor neuron pathology due to multiple sclerosis, spinal cord injury, and stroke is often painful and disabling. Muscle spasm and pain may be due to local mechanical injury including low back and neck pain, tension headache, and myofascial pain. There is limited evidence in this area but drugs used include baclofen and benzodiazepines. Botulinum toxin injected locally has been used to relax specific spastic muscles.

## 11.5 **Route and timing of administration**

### 11.5.1 **Oral**

Oral dosing is the mainstay of treatment in conscious patients with intact swallowing mechanisms for mild to moderate acute pain as well as for severe pain of long duration. Most analgesics undergo passive absorption which is largely unaltered with age.

### 11.5.2 **Topical**

Systemic analgesia is often given for a localized pain condition where a local effect is required but the risk of systemic side effects exists. There is much scepticism amongst doctors with regard to the use of topically applied analgesics, yet many patients use and appear to derive benefit from these preparations. Controlled trials of topical NSAIDs do confirm an analgesic effect; however, some of this may be due to systemic absorption and hence there remains a risk of systemic side effects. Preparations available for topical use include NSAID-containing gels, lidocaine in creams and patches, capsaicin, and topical nitrates, all of which are reported to relieve symptoms of musculoskeletal pain. In a few studies, morphine applied directly to painful ulcers and also to oral mucositis has been shown to give significant pain relief. Nitrates have been shown to be useful in painful anal fissure and also in thrombophlebitis and pain post-sclerotherapy. Whilst the evidence for these topical treatments is limited and they are not widely used in clinical practice, it is worth considering these treatments in the elderly with contraindications to or side effects from systemic therapy.

### 11.5.3 **Transdermal**

Transdermal fentanyl patches in the elderly have been shown to be effective with fewer opioid side effects and high levels of patient compliance. Most studies have looked at pain due to cancer and osteoporotic fractures. Buprenorphine patches are also available. Time to effect is prolonged as is persistent effect after removal due to its long half-life. It has a side effect profile similar to other opioids.

### 11.5.4 **Local and regional anaesthesia**

Techniques and drugs used in local and regional anaesthesia have been discussed elsewhere in this book. The effect of age on the plasma concentration of local anaesthetics after epidural administration is controversial. Some studies show that age does not affect peak plasma concentrations of lidocaine or bupivacaine or the extent of sensory anaesthesia. Other studies show a marked decrease in clearance and a moderate increase in half-life of epidural bupivacaine, suggesting that more extensive accumulation occurs in older patients with continuous epidural infusion. Anatomical changes in the epidural space and increased surface area for absorption contribute to higher plasma peak concentrations of local anaesthetics in the elderly.

Following spinal anaesthesia, the duration of blockade is prolonged in the elderly due to decreased blood flow and therefore decreased absorption in the vessels surrounding the subarachnoid space. Intrathecal morphine provides effective analgesia after pelvic and lower limb surgery; however, in the elderly the dose should be reduced to avoid adverse effects.

After epidural injection, the spread of anaesthetic agent is more extensive in the elderly so smaller volumes are needed to cover the same amount of dermatomes as in younger patients. Epidural anaesthesia with a local anaesthetic combined with an opioid provides better pain relief and improved post-operative outcome compared with systemic opioids. Studies of continuous epidural anaesthesia following knee and colon surgery show improved pain scores and improved early rehabilitation.

Peripheral nerve plexus block is useful in elderly patients with upper limb trauma as an alternative to general anaesthesia.

### 11.5.5 **PCA**

Patient-controlled analgesia (PCA) in the form of intravenous opiates, usually morphine or fentanyl, can be very useful in elderly patients. The use of PCA is limited to those with sufficient cognitive ability to understand how to use it, and, in addition, some elderly patients are also unwilling or unable to use it. For those who can, studies show that they self-administer less opiate than younger patients but report comparable pain relief and high satisfaction. There is a lower incidence of confusion, respiratory depression, and sleep disturbance in patients using PCA versus those being given boluses of intramuscular, subcutaneous, or intravenous opioids. Use also enables earlier rehabilitation and recovery.

## 11.6 **Acute pain syndromes in the elderly**

Pain management of most conditions should be based on the analgesic ladder, starting with the weakest drug at the lowest doses possible, increasing and adding stronger agents till pain is adequately relieved and using non-opioids as co-analgesics aiming to minimize the amount of opioid required. Where pain is known to be severe, common sense should prevail and starting at the bottom of the ladder is clearly inappropriate.

### 11.6.1 **Post-operative**

Pain control immediately after major surgery in the elderly should be managed similarly as in younger patients, with opiates as the mainstay of treatment. The issues already discussed in this chapter need to be considered and close monitoring and dose adjustment applied. If patients are deemed appropriate for PCA this should be used. Epidural and spinal blocks should be considered if PCA is not possible. PRN bolus dosing with or without regular background dosing should be avoided due to fluctuations in plasma concentrations and therefore more periods of overdosing and underdosing. The elderly are also less likely to request PRN drugs and may be left in pain as a result. Fentanyl patches are a very useful non-invasive option to achieve a steady state.

### 11.6.2 **Acute fractures**

Whether surgically or conservatively managed, acute limb fractures are a common cause of severe acute pain in the elderly. Pain management should be addressed in the same way as the post-operative patient. Nerve plexus block should be considered in upper limb fracture and intercostal nerve block in rib fractures.

Vertebral collapse fractures secondary to osteoporosis or tumour infiltration are common and extremely painful for a number of reasons. Acute bone fracture pain is expected and can be treated as above and resolves after a few weeks. There may be persistent pain from ligament strain or facet joint irritation. Neuropathic pain can occur in a dermatomal distribution if intercostal nerves are compressed. If lower thoracic vertebrae are affected, then the pain may be confused with abdominal visceral pain.

### 11.6.3 **Neuropathic pain**

In addition to intercostal nerve pain, neuropathic pain can occur in postherpetic neuralgia, diabetic neuropathy, trigeminal neuralgia, cervical and lumbar radiculopathy, and spinal stenosis. Anti-epileptic drugs as discussed earlier can be useful in all of these conditions, often in combination with opioids or non-opioid analgesics. Postherpetic neuralgia may also respond to sympathetic nerve block, topical capsaicin, or lidocaine and TENS.

### 11.6.4 **Stroke**

Stroke can cause pain by a number of different means. A hemiparetic shoulder can be extremely painful due to muscle spasticity, adhesive capsulitis, or shoulder–hand syndrome, all of which can be avoided by early active rehabilitation. Glenohumeral joint dislocation can occur spontaneously or accidentally be caused by a carer helping the patient up by pulling on the affected limb. The flaccid limb also has an increased risk of shoulder dislocation.

Thalamic pain syndrome involves hemianaesthesia, sensory ataxia, and sometimes choreoathetosis. This can be treated with carbamazepine or phenytoin. Central nervous system damage is also thought to lower the pain threshold, and pain seems to be more common in stroke patients with sensory impairment. Antidepressant medications can also be used in post-stroke pain as they have an effect on pain perception independent of their antidepressant effect.

# References

Abbey J, Piller N, De Bellis A *et al* (2004). The Abbey Pain Scale: a 1-minute numerical indicator for people with end-stage dementia. *International Journal of Palliative Nursing*, **10**, 6–13.

Aubrun F (2005). Management of postoperative analgesia in elderly patients. *Regional Anesthesia and Pain Medicine*, **30**, 363–79.

Buffum M and Buffum JC (2000). Nonsteroidal anti-inflammatory drugs in the elderly. *Pain Management Nursing*, **1**, 40–50.

Closs SJ, Barr B, and Briggs M (2004). Cognitive status and analgesic provision in nursing home residents. *British Journal of General Practice*, **54**, 919–21.

Cunningham C (2006). Managing pain in patients with dementia in hospital. *Nursing Standard*, **20**, 54–8.

Grimley Evans J and Franklin Williams T (eds) (2004). *Oxford Textbook of Geriatric Medicine*, 2nd edn. Oxford University Press, Oxford.

Hartnell NR, Flanagan PS, MacKinnon NJ, and Bakowsky VS (2004). Use of gastrointestinal preventive therapy among elderly persons receiving antiarthritic agents in Nova Scotia, Canada. *The American Journal of Geriatric Pharmacotherapy*, **2**, 171–80.

Kovach CR, Weissman DE, Griffe J, Matson S, Muchka S (1999). Assessment and treatment of discomfort for people with late-stage dementia. *J of Pain and Symptom Management*, **18**, 412–9.

McCleane G and Smith H (eds) (2006). *Clinical Management of the Elderly Patient in Pain*. The Haworth Medical Press, New York.

McLeskey CH (ed.) (1997). *Geriatric Anesthesiology*. Williams and Wilkins, Baltimore, MD.

Muravchick S (1997). *Geroanesthesia, Principles for Management of the Elderly Patient*. Mosby, St. Louis, MO.

Porter FL, Malhotra KM, Wolf CM, Morris JC, Miller JP, and Smith MC (1996). Dementia and response to pain in the elderly. *Pain*, **68**, 413–21.

Schuler M, Njoo N, Hestermann M, Oster P, and Hauer K (2004). Acute and chronic pain in geriatrics: clinical characteristics of pain and the influence of cognition. *Pain Medicine*, **5**, 253–62.

Vaurio LE, Sands LP, Wang Y, Mullen EA, and Leung JM (2006). Postoperative delirium: the importance of pain and pain management. *Anesthesia & Analgesia*, **102**, 1267–73.

Zwakhalen SM, Hamers JP, Abu-Saad HH, and Berger MP (2006). Pain in elderly people with severe dementia: a systematic review of behavioural pain-assessment tools. *BMC Geriatrics*, **6**, 3.

# Chapter 12

# Acute pain in pregnancy

John F.R. Dick

## Key points

- Labour pain can be severe, and relieving this pain can reduce physiological stress on mother and baby.
- Epidural and spinal analgesia is by far the most effective modality.
- Epidurals do not increase the likelihood of Caesarean delivery.
- Entonox is the next best choice for labour analgesia.
- Intravenous opioids, especially pethidine, have very little analgesic effect and cause sedation as well as other negative effects on the mother and baby.
- Transcutaneous electrical nerve stimulation has a limited role confined to early labour.

## 12.1 Pain of labour

Most women rate the pain of labour as severe or the worse imaginable. Only a few per cent report mild pain in childbirth. Labour for the first time is usually more painful than in subsequent confinements, and it is invariably of longer duration (median 14hr). Dysmenorrhoea and low social status are also associated with higher labour pain scores. Peripartum factors that predispose to more severe pain include duration of labour and artificial induction or acceleration of labour.

To accurately assess this pain, it is important that the mother scores this herself (as opioid sedation may mask a high pain score to the observer), and does so contemporaneously as the memory of pain fades consistently after the birth.

In the context of labour, pain relief is not just humane but can also reduce the associated physiological stress that can lead to maternal and foetal acidosis.

### 12.1.1 Neuroanatomy

Afferent nerve impulses from the uterus travel in A and C fibres along with sympathetic nerves and enter the spinal cord at T11 and

T12 (sometimes T10 and L1). Pain from the cervix, vagina, and perineum are transmitted via the pudendal nerves to spinal cord roots S2, S3, and S4. These fibres may be inhibited presynaptically by inhibitory neurones and opiate receptors. Visceral pain is referred to its corresponding dermatome, so that during the first stage labour pain is often localized to the lower abdomen and during the second stage more pain is felt in the perineal region. In one study, epidural blockade of T10–L1 nerve roots removed pain from the first stage of labour completely for 7 out of 11 subjects, but 4 subjects complained of pain at the pudendal nerve region (S2–4) from 8cm onwards.

### 12.1.2 **Rationale for level of epidural insertion**

The rationale for choosing the vertebral level of epidural insertion for labour analgesia is to choose a point midway between T11/12 and S2/3/4 that will eventually lead to the blockade of both nerve root sites to cover the first and second stages of labour. Also in the event of an operative block being required for Caesarean section (T4–S5), a suitable midpoint for the injection of solution must be used. Thus, the mid to lower lumbar spaces are normally used (e.g., L2/3, L3/4, L4/5). A second advantage is that the spinal cord should have terminated by L1/2, making cord or nerve damage less likely in the unlikely event of a dural tap, and that these interspaces are often the simplest to approach.

### 12.1.3 **Non-pharmacological analgesia**

The appeal of minimizing interventions in labour is self-evident; hence, the popularity of non-pharmacological pain-relieving techniques. These can be divided into two methods: psychological and physical.

#### 12.1.3.1 *Psychological methods*

Apart from anticipated pain, other stressors such as the possibility of complications surrounding delivery for mother and baby may well increase anxiety about labour. Thus, antenatal education covering the whole childbirth process and specifically labour pain and the options for pain management is crucial, particularly for primiparas.

*Relaxation techniques* include simple breathing techniques as well as muscle relaxation exercises can be used.

*Self-hypnosis* appears to work in well-motivated individuals. Both techniques are more effective if learnt and practised in the antenatal period.

*Supporting person* may be a partner, friend, midwife, or Doula and is thought to have a positive effect on a variety of outcomes including a reduction in analgesic requirements.

### 12.1.3.2 *Physical methods*

*Alternative analgesia* using aromatherapy and reflexology are also popular but require a practitioner to be present.

*Water baths* probably work by aiding relaxation, increasing endogenous opioid secretions, and may also work in a way similar to transcutaneous electrical nerve stimulation (TENS). Satisfaction is high but there is little evidence to suggest any reduction in pain scores. It is not possible to continuously monitor the foetal heart in the birth pool. The pool is also unsafe for mothers with intravenous infusions running or continuous maternal monitoring.

*TENS* is thought to work by stimulating A fibres in the posterior primary rami, which inhibit transmitter release from A and C fibres that transmit pain from the uterus. Thus, when placed over A fibres at T10–L1 they may reduce early labour pain. Pains associated with the later stages of labour are often referred to the dermatomes of S2–4 and are poorly blocked by TENS. Randomized controlled trials of TENS versus dummy TENS have shown no difference in pain intensity and similar requirements for supplementary analgesia in both groups. TENS appears to be safe for the foetus and has no significant side effects for the mother.

*Acupuncture* is uncommonly used for labour analgesia in the United Kingdom. Acupuncture needles are inserted at various points in the body corresponding to the same points used for the treatment of dysmenorrhoea. Needles may be left *in situ* or manipulated by rotation or stimulated electrically. No randomized trials exist to confirm efficacy. One study, performed by a professor of the Chinese College of Acupuncture in Hong Kong, was abandoned as 90% of volunteers for manual and electrical acupuncture failed to gain adequate analgesia. However, maternal satisfaction rates remain relatively high using this technique. The treatments require a number of sessions before labour and are expensive. No adverse effects on mother, labour, and child are reported but there is a lack of suitable trials on the subject.

*Water blocks* consist of intradermal injections of 0.1mL sterile water in four spots over the sacrum that produces a transient burning sensation. The mode of action may be similar to that of TENS. Some efficacy over placebo using saline has been demonstrated but there was no reduction in the need for additional analgesia.

### 12.1.4 **Pharmacological methods**

#### 12.1.4.1 *Systemic opioids*

These drugs have been used in labour since Greek and Roman times. There was a fashion for their use in large doses combined with hyoscine in the early 1900s to produce 'twilight sleep' in labour. However, the side effects, which included maternal and foetal respiratory depression, were severe and the technique has been abandoned since the 1930s.

*Pethidine (known as meperidine in some countries)*

This is the most widely used opioid in labour. Midwives in the United Kingdom are allowed to administer up to 150mg intramuscularly to a labouring woman without medical prescription. When given systemically pethidine acts principally upon μ and κ receptors in the brain rather than the spinal cord. Pethidine causes sedation well before adequate analgesia is achieved. A degree of sedation probably detracts from the experience of birth for the mother. Oversedation is frankly dangerous for mother and foetus. In addition, pethidine increases nausea and vomiting and reduces gastric emptying, which is significant if emergency general anaesthesia is required to deliver the baby or manage haemorrhage.

The effect of pethidine on the neonates may be explained by a high placental transfer rate, the possibility of ion trapping in an acidotic foetus and the prolonged half-life of the sedative metabolite norpethidine (62hr) in the foetus. Neonatal respiratory depression is well documented after the administration of pethidine to the mother and is worst 3hr after a dose, and with repeated dosing. Furthermore, babies may develop subtle neurobehavioural changes compared to non-opioid receiving mothers, and may take longer to establish breastfeeding. These effects on the neonate may be reversed with naloxone.

*Morphine*

Probably no better than pethidine in reducing pain scores and also profoundly sedative. With this sedative effect in mind, standardized morphine patient-controlled analgesias (PCAs) are offered to mothers who have suffered an intrauterine death and are encouraged to deliver the dead foetus.

*Diamorphine*

Less frequently used compared to pethidine but gaining in popularity. This may have advantages over pethidine in terms of reduced vomiting, a longer duration of action, and more favourable 1min Apgar scores.

*Fentanyl*

Produces similar analgesia to pethidine when given intravenously, but maternal nausea and sedation are reduced. It has been associated with transient decreases in the foetal heart rate.

*Remifentanil*

Is a pure μ-agonist with fast onset and with a reliable and fast offset (context-sensitive half-life of 3min). These characteristics may make remifentanil an ideal patient-controlled analgesic in labour. Remifentanil produces a greater reduction in VAS scores in labour compared to pethidine and entonox, but produces similar degrees of sedation to other opioids. Pruritus is another side effect, although rarely requires treatment. The dose has been evaluated at between 0.2mcg/kg and 0.8mcg/kg and the lockout period is normally set to 2min. Remifentanil

PCA was not associated with significantly adverse effects in a trial of 50 parturients that specifically assessed maternal and neonatal well-being.

A recent survey of UK maternity units showed that remifentanil PCA is becoming increasingly available. It is hoped that this may be a suitable analgesic for those mothers in whom epidural analgesia is contraindicated.

There is concern that the time to peak effect means that remifentanil fails to provide adequate analgesia for the early part of the contraction.

### 12.1.4.2 *Nitrous oxide*

Is an inhalational agent that has analgesic properties at sub-anaesthetic doses. It was first used in labour in the 1880s. Entonox®, a 50/50 mixture of nitrous oxide and oxygen, was developed by Tunstall in 1961. This mixture has been chosen so as to balance the analgesic effect against the increasing sedation associated with higher concentrations of nitrous oxide. The gas is available in nearly all maternity suites in the United Kingdom as cylinders and piped direct to wall outlets. A demand valve and face mask is commonly used to deliver the gas. Nitrous oxide is extremely insoluble and reaches an effective arterial concentration within 15–20sec and produces maximum analgesia at around 45–60sec. Thus, timing of inspirations with the very beginning of a contraction is essential.

In terms of efficacy, nitrous oxide mixtures have significant analgesic effect in labour when compared to oxygen or air in all but one study. However, it rarely offers complete analgesia and a significant proportion will not find it helpful. In the National Birthday Trust survey (1993), Entonox® was helpful in the relief of pain in a higher proportion than intramuscular pethidine (43% vs. 28%) and was second only to epidural analgesia.

Common maternal side effects include dizziness and a drunken feeling, which may progress to marked sedation. Memory of the labour process may be impaired. Nausea and vomiting are quite common (up to 20%). Fortunately, nitrous oxide does not appear to affect the progress or duration of labour and has no known clinical effects on the foetus or newborn.

In summary, nitrous oxide is a cheap, widely available and relatively safe compound that may offer satisfactory analgesia in labour.

## 12.2 Regional anaesthesia

### 12.2.1 *Epidural analgesia*

This involves the insertion of a fine plastic catheter into the epidural space and the delivery of analgesic mixtures to affect analgesia of nearby nerve roots. The mid to lower lumbar interspaces are most commonly used for reasons described earlier. It is also possible to deliver epidural analgesia via the caudal route (usually, a single injection through the sacrococcygeal membrane) to block the sacral nerve roots in the event of an instrumental delivery.

The advantages of this form of analgesia are manyfold. It provides the best analgesia in terms of pain scores (see Figure 12.1) and can reduce the pain of contractions completely. When well performed, epidural analgesia reduces maternal catecholamine release and this improves placental perfusion.

The technique results in far less systemic spread of drug compared with intravenous opioids resulting in less maternal sedation and improved neonatal Apgar scores. An epidural block may be extended to provide analgesia and anaesthesia for instrumental delivery as well as Caesarean section. It is this last fact that has significantly reduced the rate of general anaesthesia for emergency Caesarean section, which has probably made the greatest contribution to the reduction in maternal mortality attributed to anaesthesia. Finally, epidural solutions will also produce a blockade of the sympathetic nervous system, which is useful to reduce maternal blood pressure in pre-eclampsia.

The disadvantages are that it requires expertise to perform and run an epidural service. Strict maternal and foetal monitoring is required with each epidural injection. At best, it is likely to take 20–30min after requesting epidural analgesia before the block begins to work. There is a small but significant degree of morbidity associated with the process (dural puncture headache occurring around 1% of cases). There is a small increase in the duration of labour and there is also a small rise in instrumental delivery rate. However, epidural analgesia does not appear to increase the rate of Caesarean section.

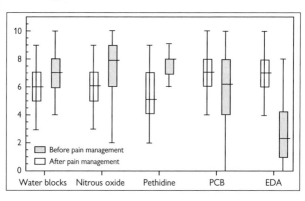

**Figure 12.1** Visual pain scores for 833 Finnish women (71% primiparas) averaged over the whole labour. Note that only epidural analgesia (EDA) resulted in significant reductions in pain scores. PCB, paracervical block.

Visual pain scale scores (0–10) *before* and *after* pain management in the first stage of labour in the various pain relief groups. Minimum, lower (25%) quartile, median, upper (75%) quartile, maximum.

The main indications for commencing an epidural infusion in labour are maternal request. There are also situations in which epidural analgesia is strongly advised, for example, pre-eclampsia or where there is a high likelihood of a labour progressing to operative delivery.

### 12.2.1.1 *Epidural solutions*

Most units in the United Kingdom now use a mixture of bupivacaine in low concentration (e.g., 0.1%) with fentanyl in low dose (2mcg/mL). Previously, stronger solutions of local anaesthetic were used alone but these were associated with an unacceptable degree of motor block. By using combinations of local anaesthetic and opioid, lower doses may be used which results in a block that is more targeted for the sensory nerves. This will allow most mothers to be 'mobile' with their epidural. Another advantage of these lower doses is that they are safer if inadvertently injected intravenously.

The commonest method of delivery is by bolus dose through the epidural catheter delivered by the anaesthetist or midwife with a minimum time interval before subsequent dosing. An increasingly popular technique is to allow patient-controlled boluses via a pump that allows more maternal control although the patient may find the presence of the pump restricting. Epidural solutions can also be delivered by continuous infusion which again requires a pump. Unfortunately, when compared to the bolus technique, this method is associated with the administration of greater volumes of solution and higher degrees of motor block. It has been demonstrated that giving regular automated boluses via a pump (rather than on maternal request) produces better analgesia (less breakthrough pain) and greater patient satisfaction compared to an identical hourly dose run as an infusion.

### 12.2.2 **Spinal**

Subarachnoid injection of local anaesthetic and opioid solutions may also be used for labour analgesia and may take the form of a single-shot spinal or combined spinal epidural. The advantages of a spinal injection over epidural are quicker onset of analgesia, but this has to be balanced with the fact that dural puncture is associated with a small but important rate of dural puncture headache (reduced with small non-cutting needles). Spinal injection during labour can be accompanied by epidural insertion (combined spinal epidural), which has the advantage of a faster onset of analgesia from the spinal component and leaving an epidural catheter in place for subsequent infusions.

## 12.3 **Non-labour pain in pregnancy**

Abdominal pain in pregnancy can be a result of labour, premature or timely, or causes unrelated to the pregnancy.

Labour pain is intermittent, associated with tightening and contractions, it is accompanied by shortening of the cervix and engagement of the foetal head.

### 12.3.1 **Obstetric causes of abdominal pain**

In addition to the commencement of labour, number of other obstetric events can cause an onset of acute pain. In early pregnancy, ectopic pregnancy and miscarriage can both present as abdominal pain. Later in pregnancy, the sudden onset of pain may be associated with placental abruption. Throughout the pregnancy, pain related to ovarian cyst or intrauterine fibroids may be a feature. Epigastric and right upper quadrant pain is associated with pre-eclampsia, HELLP syndrome, and fatty liver.

### 12.3.2 **Non-obstetric causes of abdominal pain**

Acute pain from any other cause can occur in pregnancy. Constipation is common in pregnancy and can cause significant pain. Also, infection, appendicitis, and renal colic can all occur. Thrombosis of the iliac vessels is uncommon but has been recorded in pregnancy. Metabolic disturbances such as hypercalcaemia may cause abdominal pain.

### 12.3.3 **Pharmacological management of acute pain in pregnancy**

Treatment of acute pain in pregnancy is limited by the potential for maternal–foetal transfer of the drug and subsequent effects on the foetus.

*Opioids* cross the placenta and can be detected in the amniotic fluid from 12 weeks of gestation. Whilst short-term use of opioids for acute pain during pregnancy has not been associated with either teratogenic effects or significant impairment of the foetus, chronic opioid use during the pregnancy results in addiction in the newborn that will require specialist neonatal management.

#### 12.3.3.1 *Non-steroidal anti-inflammatory drugs*

These should be avoided during pregnancy. This is particularly so during the third trimester. Non-steroidal anti-inflammatory drugs (NSAIDs) can suppress foetal renal function producing oligohydramnos, and also the use of NSAIDs in the mother may produce premature closure of the ductus arteriosis.

#### 12.3.3.2 *Paracetamol*

Paracetamol is safe in pregnancy and is the analgesic of choice.

# References

Abe N (1980). Clinical analysis of the pain pathways of labor. *Nippon Sanka Fujinka Gakkai Zasshi*, **32**, 6–10.

Carstoniu J, Levytam S, Norman P, Daley D, Katz J, and Sandler AN (1994). Nitrous oxide in early labor. Safety and analgesic efficacy assessed by a double-blind, placebo-controlled study. *Anesthesiology*, **80**, 30–5.

Fairlie FM, Marshall L, Walker JJ, and Elbourne D (1999). Intramuscular opioids for maternal pain relief in labour: a randomised controlled trial comparing pethidine with diamorphine. *British Journal of Obstetrics and Gynaecology*, **106**, 1181–7.

Lim Y, Sia AT, and Ocampo C (2005). Automated regular boluses for epidural analgesia: a comparison with continuous infusion. *International Journal of Obstetric Anesthesia*, **14**, 305–9.

Melzack R, Kinch R, Dobkin P, Lebrun M, and Taenzer P (1984). Severity of labour pain: influence of physical as well as psychologic variables. *Canadian Medical Association Journal*, **130**, 579–84.

Norvell KT, Gaston-Johansson F, and Fridh G (1987). Remembrance of labor pain: how valid are retrospective pain measurements? *Pain*, **31**, 77–86.

National Birthday Trust survey (1993).

Ranta P, Jouppila P, Spalding M, Kangas-Saarela T, Hollmén A, and Jouppila R (1994). Parturients' assessment of water blocks, pethidine, nitrous oxide, paracervical and epidural blocks in labour. *International Journal of Obstetric Anesthesia*, **14**, 193–8.

Saravanakumar K, Garstang JS, and Hasan K (2007). Intravenous patient-controlled analgesia for labour: a survey of UK practice. *International Journal of Obstetric Anesthesia*, **16**, 221–5.

Thomas IL, Tyle V, Webster J, and Neilson A (1988). An evaluation of transcutaneous electrical nerve stimulation for pain relief in labour. *The Australian and New Zealand Journal of Obstetrics and Gynaecology*, **28**, 182–9.

Volikas I, Butwick A, Wilkinson C, Pleming A, and Nicholson G (2005). Maternal and neonatal side-effects of remifentanil patient-controlled analgesia in labour. *British Journal of Anaesthesia*, **95**, 504–9.

Wallis L, Shnider SM, Palahniuk RJ, and Spivey HT (1974). An evaluation of acupuncture analgesia in obstetrics. *Anesthesiology*, **41**, 596–601.

# Chapter 13

# Acute pain in cancer

James A. Smart

> **Key points**
>
> - Pain in patients with cancer occurs because of a variety of different causes and has both nociceptive and neuropathic pain components.
> - It is essential that a thorough assessment of the pain is carried out in order to institute appropriate treatment.
> - Whilst the WHO Pain Ladder is a good place to start, there are many other treatments available to treat pain in cancer.
> - Any pharmacological or interventional treatment will be more successful if appropriate psychological support is provided.

## 13.1 Background

Each year approximately 250 000 people in the United Kingdom are diagnosed with cancer. Half of these people suffer from breast, bowel, lung, or prostatic carcinomas. Of these patients, about 30% will have pain when they are diagnosed and between 60% and 90% will have pain if the disease becomes advanced.

There have been huge improvements in the treatment of pain due to cancer. These improvements are largely because of the introduction of the World Health Organization's 'Pain Ladder' in 1986. It is intended for use around the world in both developed and developing nations. The ladder was designed as a simple and cheap method of controlling the pain of over 80% of patients with advanced cancer, using pharmacological means.

In the United Kingdom, we have access to classes of drugs and interventional procedures that compliment the WHO Pain Ladder. These treatments give improved analgesia and quality of life to cancer sufferers.

### 13.1.1 Types of pain

Pain can be usefully subdivided according to its cause, either the physiological nociceptive pain or the pathological neuropathic pain.

Nociceptive pain is perceived in response to tissue damage and inflammation.

Neuropathic pain, however, can after damage to a peripheral or central nerve or after prolonged exposure of a nociceptive neurone to a painful stimulus. The subsequent aberrant somatosensory processing is perceived as pain. Neuropathic pain may be described as an unfamiliar or strange sensation, often as a burning sensation or a brief shooting pain with an electrical shock-like quality.

Whilst nociceptive pain may well have a neuropathic component, it is still useful to differentiate between the two as the pharmacological treatments can be quite different.

### 13.1.2 Causes of pain due to cancer

Pain in patients with cancer is usually caused by either the growth of the tumour itself or secondary to the treatments and investigations undergone.

Tumour growth may cause pain directly or indirectly. Directly, there may be associated tissue damage by local invasion of tissues and nerves or pain caused by metastasis, for example, to bone causing osteolysis, pathological fractures, and nerve compression or to lung causing pleural irritation. Indirectly, the effects of the tumour can cause pain as a result of raised intracranial pressure, lymphoedema, or muscular spasm.

Post-operative pain and post-investigation pain may be a factor in the treatment course of many patients. This pain is usually nociceptive but may well have a neuropathic pain component. If the patient is on high doses of opiates or other analgesics, then these should, if possible, be continued throughout the post-operative period. Additional post-operative analgesia should be prescribed for the pain of the operation. The local pain team may want to give advice on prescribing in these situations.

### 13.1.3 Assessment

It is essential that a full assessment of the patient's pain be carried out when the symptoms first present. This assessment must be reviewed if there is an acute change in the severity of the pain (Table 13.1).

- The effect of the pain on the patient should also be recorded, for example, effects on sleep, mood, and day to day activities
- Aspirations should be elicited and realistic goals set
- Using tools such as the Short Form McGill Pain Questionnaire and visual analogue scales or verbal rating scales can help assessment
- Physical examination is usually essential to correctly identify the cause of the pain and institute correct treatment
- Radiological investigations often help in determining whether interventional procedures will be helpful and possible.

## Table 13.1 Pain assessment

- Severity
- Duration
- Quality
- Nature
- Variation (e.g., night and day, week to week, etc.)
- Site and radiation
- Exacerbating/reliving factors
- Treatments tried (effective and ineffective)

## 13.2 Pharmacological treatments

### 13.2.1 The WHO Pain Ladder

The WHO Pain Ladder is a simple and cheap yet effective method of controlling pain in cancer using widely available drugs (Figure 13.1). The patient's starts at the level of the ladder corresponding to his/her pain, that is, if the patient is suffering from severe pain then they will start at the top of the ladder with a strong opioid and non-steroidal anti-inflammatory drug (NSAID) ± adjuvant.

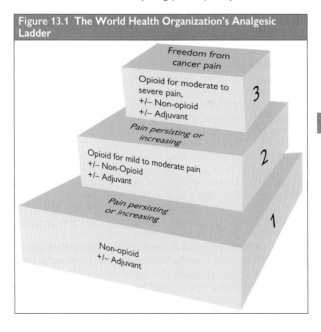

Figure 13.1 The World Health Organization's Analgesic Ladder

Freedom from cancer pain

Opioid for moderate to severe pain,
+/– Non-opioid
+/– Adjuvant   3

Pain persisting or increasing

Opioid for mild to moderate pain
+/– Non-Opioid
+/– Adjuvant   2

Pain persisting or increasing

Non-opioid
+/– Adjuvant   1

### 13.2.2 **Paracetamol**

Paracetamol provides a synergistic analgesic effect with NSAIDs and opiates when given regularly. Paracetamol works as an anti-inflammatory on the cyclooxygenase (COX) system although its action seems to be limited to the central rather than peripheral nervous system. It has few side effects although it is highly toxic when taken in overdose.

### 13.2.3 **NSAIDs**

NSAIDs work via the COX pathway preventing prostaglandin synthesis. They have marked peripheral anti-inflammatory effects making them very useful as analgesics, although their use is limited by their side effects. Using a proton pump inhibitor such as omeprazole may reduce gastrointestinal side effects. This is often effective for bony pain, where traditionally a combination of aspirin and an opiate have been used very effectively. NSAIDs differ in their potency in this type of pain. For example, dexketoprofen has been shown to be more effective than keterolac in bony pain.

### 13.2.4 **Opioids**

#### 13.2.4.1 *Weak opioids*

Include tramadol, codeine, and dihydrocodeine and seem to offer little increased benefit of one over another. If one is poorly tolerated, then it is worth trying the alternatives.

#### 13.2.4.2 *Strong opioids*

Any opiate should be introduced by gradual titration to minimize side effects. They can be given by a variety of routes although the default route should be oral (Table 13.2).

Morphine will probably be the first strong opioid that a patient will try but there are other alternatives that are also widely available. Morphine is often given as a sustained release preparation with immediate release. Morphine prescribed for breakthrough pain. Breakthrough pain is a sudden increase in the level continuous pain which 'breaks through' the regular analgesia prescribed. The dose of breakthrough analgesia should be 20% of the daily regular morphine dose.

While it may seem slightly illogical, there is good evidence showing that if morphine is an ineffective analgesic or if the side effects are intolerable then switching to another opioid may well provide better relief from the pain and/or adverse effects.

As tolerance to one opioid develops, it may become necessary to change to an alternative opiate. This 'opiate rotation' is widely used although not universally regarded as useful. When rotating opiates, the dose of the original opiate should be converted to the equivalent dose of the new opiate. This equipotent dose should then be reduced by 30–50%, as an equipotent conversion will sometimes cause an

**Table 13.2 Opiate conversion**

| Oral opioid (dose in mg per 24hr) | | Subcutaneous infusion of opioid (syringe driver dose in mg per 24hr) | | | | Opioid by patch (dose in mcg/hr, 72 hourly patches) | |
|---|---|---|---|---|---|---|---|
| Morphine | Oxycodone | Morphine | Diamorphine | Oxycodone | Alfentanil | Fentanyl | Buprenorphine |
| | 1/2 oral morphine dose | 1/2 oral morphine dose | 1/3 oral morphine dose | 1/2 oral oxycodone dose | 1/10 diamorphine equivalent | See manufacturer's charts for equivalence—reproduced here | |
| 20 | 10 | 10 | 5 | 5 | N/A | N/A | N/A |
| 40 | 20 | 20 | 15 | 10 | 2 | (12) | 35 |
| 90 | 45 | 45 | 30 | 20 | 3 | 25 | 52.5 |
| 180 | 90 | 90 | 60 | 45 | 6 | 50 | 105 |
| 280 | 140 | 140 | 90 | 70 | 9 | 75 | 140 |
| 360 | 180 | Use alfentanil | 120 | 90 | 12 | 100 | N/A |

Opioid dose conversion chart adapted from Cancer Care Alliance Palliative Care Guidelines for the End of Life, October 2005 (www.cancercarealliance.nhs.uk). N/A, not available.

increase in side effects including respiratory depression. If necessary, the patient can compensate for the decreased dose using their break-through analgesia. The regular dose can then be increased appropriately over the next few days.

Alternative strong opioids are oxycodone, fentanyl, diamorphine, and hydromorphone.

Methadone is a difficult analgesic to use although it is widely used and can be very effective in some patients. The variability in analgesic effect and duration between patients is extensive and the plasma half-life is protracted. Its NMDA antagonist action can be useful in neuropathic types of cancer pain.

### 13.2.4.3 *Ketamine*

Ketamine has useful effects on both nociceptive and neuropathic pain. It is a competitive antagonist at the NMDA receptor preventing both physiological pain transmission and central sensitization, which are both mediated by the receptor. Ketamine also reduces the effects of opiate tolerance and has an opiate-sparing effect. The analgesic effects of ketamine can far outlast its duration in the plasma although the duration of its effects are variable.

Ketamine is usually given via the intravenous, subcutaneous or sublingual route.

Adverse effects of ketamine, which may limit its use, are acutely dysphoria and hallucinations and chronically memory impairment and behavioural changes. Most of the acute effects can be reduced by appropriate dosing and the administration of a benzodiazepine.

### 13.2.4.4 *Bisphosphonates*

Drugs that are ingested by osteoclasts inhibiting the reabsorbtion of bone. They are useful in treating pain caused by multiple myeloma and osteolytic metastasis, for examples, breast and prostatic metastasis. Patients on bisphosphonates have a reduced need for radiotherapy (indicating less pain), less pathological fractures, and a lower incidence of hypercalcaemia.

### 13.2.4.5 *Gabapentin*

Gabapentin works by blocking calcium channels in the presynaptic neurone, inhibiting vesicular transmission to the basement membrane, and therefore transmission of the nerve impulse. Gabapentin has recently been shown to decrease nociceptive pain in post-operative patients whilst also decreasing anxiety, having an opiate-sparing effect and acting as an anti-emetic.

Gabapentin has been widely used to treat neuropathic pain for 15yrs and can help reduce neuropathic and nociceptive pain in patients with cancer.

Gabapentin should be introduced slowly to prevent its most common side effects, which include diplopia, ataxia, and somnolence. If the patient is introducing the drug at home and continuing day to day activity such as driving, then an increase of 300mg per week is appropriate. This titration can be accelerated if they are an inpatient.

Pregabalin is a drug in the same group, which has two advantages over gabapentin. It seems to have a faster onset of action and also has a more predictable bioavailability (the bioavailability of gabapentin decreases with dose).

### 13.2.4.6 *Other anticonvulsants and antidepressants*

Carbamazepine, amitriptyline, and levetiracetam, all have a place in treating the neuropathic component of pain.

Clonazepam also has a role if muscular spasms are causing significant problems.

### 13.2.4.7 *Cannabis*

There are currently strict restrictions on prescribing cannabinoids in the United Kingdom, although they have been shown to reduce pain caused by cancer.

Endogenous cannabinoids are found in the post-synaptic membrane and travel across the synapse to the presynaptic receptors to reduce transmission of neuronal impulses. Physiologically, they act as a break on the normal stresses we encounter and switch us into 'relaxation mode'. They are among the most widely expressed receptors in the body and are important mediators in pain transmission.

Sativex® is the only cannabinoid available for prescription at present and only under licence from the Home Office. It is formulated as a mixture of delta-9-tetrahydrocannabinol (Δ9THC) (active component) and cannabidiol (which modulates the psychotropic effects of the THC).

### 13.2.4.8 *Lidocaine and mexiletine*

Neurones in patients with neuropathic pain have increased the expression of tetrodotoxin-resistant sodium channels that are blocked by lidocaine and mexiletine. Their effect is, therefore, more on the neuropathic pain component.

They are associated with serious side effects such as arrhythmias, which may limit their use in high doses. The toxic plasma levels of lidocaine are very well recorded and staying within prescribing limits will generally avoid any adverse events.

## 13.3 **Non-pharmacological treatments**

### 13.3.1 **Radiotherapy**

Radiotherapy has been shown to be effective in reducing or eliminating the pain from bone metastases in 70% of patients. Pain from bony metastases can be eliminated in just under 30% of patients and reduced by 50% in over 40% of patients. The full analgesic effects may take some weeks to develop although the effects are usually apparent in 7–10 days. Radiotherapy can also be used to treat pain caused by soft tissue tumours and metastases (e.g., mesothelioma).

Radiotherapy is usually delivered via an external beam although if the metastases are widespread then irradiation using radioactive isotopes may be considered. The effects of external beam therapy are usually apparent much faster than isotope therapy. The doses of radiation are usually low and side effects are often minimal and limited to tiredness post-treatment.

### 13.3.2 **Chemotherapy**

Chemotherapy may be used to treat pain secondary to cancer although its use is usually limited by its side effects; however, in advanced disease it is worth considering.

### 13.3.3 **Interventional procedures**

There are many interventional procedures that we can utilize to alleviate the pain of cancer, ranging from epidural blockade to the insertion of indwelling catheters next to single nerves or plexuses. Most blocks will require either fluoroscopic, computed tomography, or ultrasound guidance.

Neurolytic coeliac plexus blockade using alcohol can provide analgesia in 90% of patients and has low incidence (1%) of serious side effects.

Epidural analgesia can be profound and, if left *in situ*, long lasting. But care and use of an epidural analgesic system is complex and failure and infection are constant risks.

Plexus and specific nerve blocks are useful tools and can also provide long-lasting benefit if an indwelling catheter is inserted. The use of these blocks requires skilled staff to perform the block and provide care to maintain the therapy. Close liaison with the palliative care and hospice staff is essential.

### 13.3.4 **Psychological support**

The psychological effects of developing cancer are wide ranging. Patients can become depressed, scared, or angry. They can suffer from general anxiety or panic attacks, withdraw from their friends and family, develop sleep problems, and loose interest in food and sex. All of these problems, whilst deserving of treatment in their own right, will exacerbate any symptoms of pain and should therefore be addressed as a priority in their pain management plan.

The level of support needed will vary from patient to patient and the availability of services may also vary. The Palliative Care/Symptom Control team in your hospital will often be the most useful source of information in this area.

# References

Cancer Research UK News and Resources (year). CancerStats. Available at http://info.cancerresearchuk.org/cancerstats/incidence/?a=5441#incidence (accessed February 2010).

González P, Cabello P, Germany A, Norris B, and Contreras E (1997). Decrease of tolerance to, and physical dependence on morphine by, glutamate receptor antagonists. *European Journal of Pharmacology*, **332**, 257–62.

Ischia S, Ischia A, Polati E, and Finco G (1992). Three posterior percutaneous celiac plexus block techniques. A prospective, randomized study in 61 patients with pancreatic cancer pain. *Anesthesiology*, **76**, 534–40.

Keskinbora K, Pekel A, and Aydinli I (2007). Gabapentin and an opioid combination versus opioid alone for the management of neuropathic cancer pain: a randomized open trial. *Journal of Pain Symptom Management*, **34**, 183–9.

Leppert W and Luczak J (2005). The role of tramadol in cancer pain treatment—a review. *Supportive Care in Cancer*, **13**, 5–17.

McQuay HJ, Carroll D, and Moore RA (1997). Radiotherapy for painful bone metastases. a systematic review. *Clinical Oncology*, **9**, 150–4.

Ménigaux C, Adam F, Guignard B, Sessler DI, and Chauvin M (2005). Preoperative gabapentin decreases anxiety and improves early functional recovery from knee surgery. *Anesthesia & Analgesics*, **100**, 1394–9.

Riley J, Ross JR, Rutter D, et al. (2006). No pain relief from morphine? Individual variation in sensitivity to morphine and the need to switch to an alternative opioid in cancer patients. *Supportive Care in Cancer*, **14**, 56–64.

Ross JR, Saunders Y, Edmonds PM, Patel S, K Broadley E, and Johnston SRD (2003). Systematic review of role of bisphosphonates on skeletal morbidity in metastatic cancer. *BMJ*, **327**, 469.

Singh G and Triadafilopoulos G (2005). Appropriate choice of proton pump inhibitor therapy in the prevention and management of NSAID-related gastrointestinal damage. *International Journal of Clinical Practice*, **59**, 1210–17.

# Chapter 14

# Acute pain in haematological disorders

Ali Mofeez, Upal Hossain

## Key points

- The use of painkillers ranging from simple analgesics to strong opioids is a common feature in the acute pain management of haematological conditions.
- However, each disease also has its own specific aetiological factors for pain, requiring specific treatment.
- Haematological patients with chronic pain on long-term opioid therapy may require multidisciplinary pain management to improve quality of life and prevent chronic escalation of opioid doses.
- Intramuscular injections should be avoided in all patients.
- The use of pethidine (meperidine) is not recommended.

## 14.1 Sickle cell disease

### 14.1.1 Definition

Sickle cell disease (SCD) is a recessively inherited group of disorders involving a single-base mutation in the β-gene on chromosome 11 resulting in the production of abnormal haemoglobin (HbSS). In addition, the homozygous HbSS, other variants with considerable morbidity include HbSC and HbS/β-thalassaemia.

### 14.1.2 Pathophysiology

The abnormal Hb polymerizes when deoxygenated, causing the erythrocyte to change from its usual plate-like shape to a rigid, crescent, or sickle shape (sickle cells) with overall increased blood viscosity.

Pain is variable and is as a result of complex, not fully understood mechanisms. Vasoocclusion is the most important event for the development of acute sickle cell pain, leading to tissue damage, which initiates a series of biochemical events and cellular interactions resulting in the perception of pain. Psychological, social, cultural, and spiritual factors further influence the perception of pain.

These crises can be spontaneous or precipitated by triggers such as dehydration, infection, fatigue, emotional or physical stress, temperature change, hypoxia, menstruation, or pregnancy.

Generally, SCD patients with high-Hb levels are more likely to have frequent painful crises than those with lower Hb levels.

Patients may suffer acute painful episodes and/or more chronic long-standing pain.

### 14.1.3 **Acute painful crisis**

Acute painful crisis is the number one cause of hospital admission for patients with SCD.

There is large interindividual variability regarding frequency and severity of crises, ranging from absent or very mild to frequent, severe pain requiring hospitalization and opioid analgesia. Typically, the pain of an acute crisis is severe.

Sites of pain include bone (causing bone pain), joints (hip, knee, shoulder elbow), lungs (causing acute chest crisis), spleen (causing painful splenomegaly and splenic infarction especially in children), and the penis (causing priapism).

Acute chest syndrome presents with chest pain, cough, dyspnoea, fever, leucocytosis, and pulmonary infiltrates on CXR. This may be due to rib or lung infarction or underlying pneumonia. Those with underlying pneumonia tend to be more systemically unwell.

Sickle cell pain is primarily a nociceptive pain. But it may also have a neuropathic component with or without any obvious central or peripheral nerve injury. Trigeminal neuralgia, entrapment neuropathy, and acute demyelinating neuropathy have been described in SCD. The aetiology is uncertain but may be due to abnormal processing in the central or peripheral nervous system.

### 14.1.4 **Basic management**

Initial management should assess for treatable complications such as dehydration, anaemia, infection, priapism, or evidence of acute chest syndrome.

Therefore, fluid replacement and oxygen therapy is part of the first-line treatment. Antibiotics should be used in the appropriate setting and according to local policies.

To date, oxygen therapy has not been shown to decrease pain. Two studies showed no difference in pain duration, number of pain sites, or opioid consumption in patients treated with air or oxygen. However, it is considered good practice to include oxygen in the management of acute crises, aiming to reverse the sickling process, and increase oxygen-carrying capacity in anaemic patients.

In addition, other indications in the management of sickle patients, blood/exchange transfusions may also be considered for pain management in consultation with the haematologists. These may be useful in the acute setting (e.g., acute chest crisis) or in those with frequent, acute painful crises, aiming to reduce the rate of recurrence through a regular blood transfusion or exchange transfusion program (e.g., monthly for a period of several months).

Patients (adults and children) are often distressed and frightened during painful crisis. Thus, reassurance as well as distraction techniques may be beneficial at such times.

#### 14.1.4.1 *Analgesia*
The chosen analgesic regimen may be aided from treatment received in previous admissions. Therefore, obtaining the patient's previous medical or accident and emergency records (including analgesia records) can be very informative.

#### 14.1.4.2 *Paracetamol (acetaminophen) and NSAIDs*
Recommended for mild to moderate pain but non-steroidal anti-inflammatory drugs (NSAIDs) should be used with caution if sickling has caused renal impairment. In the acute setting, ketorolac is the only NSAID with evidence of proven benefit. Other NSAIDs such as ibuprofen and diclofenac can also be used. In general, the oral route of administration is preferred and the intramuscular route should be avoided because of the risk of abscess formation (especially with diclofenac due to the volume of injection).

In acute sickle crises, NSAIDs probably reduce opioid requirements but strong evidence is lacking.

#### 14.1.4.3 *Opioids*
Recommended for more severe pain and should be prescribed with a laxative. Morphine, fentanyl, hydromorphone, and oxycodone are the commonest opioids used. For treating acute sickle crises, the route of administration is usually intravenous (most commonly as patient-controlled analgesia [PCA] or continuous intravenous infusion). However, regular oral sustained-release opioids with readily available immediate release opioids have been shown to be equally effective and should be considered as first-line treatment unless the oral route is contraindicated. Oral opioid protocols have been shown to reduce the number of A&E visits and the frequency of hospital admissions (Friedman *et al.* 1986; Conti *et al.* 1996). Other routes of administration include transdermal and transmucosal. Historically, intramuscular injections were common practice; however, this is generally not recommended due to infection risk as well as risk of addictive behaviour (which also has been observed with the anti-emetic cyclizine).

#### 14.1.4.4 *Adjuvants*

Anticonvulsants (e.g., gabapentin) and antidepressants (e.g., amitriptyline) are used if there is a neuropathic component to the pain.

#### 14.1.4.5 *Interventions*

Regional anaesthetic procedures such as epidural analgesia, peripheral nerve blocks, or intercostal blocks have been used effectively in severe pain unresponsive to high-dose opioids, NSAIDs, and adjunctive analgesics.

### 14.1.5 **Other treatment**

Inhaled $N_2O$ (nitrous oxide) can be used for a limited period, and may provide some analgesia in the initial stages (e.g., primary care setting or in the first 60min of an acute crisis such as in an ambulance).

*Inhaled NO (nitric oxide)*: NO deficiency may be involved in the pathophysiology of vasoocclusive crises. Thus, inhaled NO may help in the treatment of painful crises.

*Arginine supplements* are also used with the aim of increasing nitric oxide levels (Morris et al. 2003).

*Corticosteroids*: A short course of high-dose Methylprednisolone may decrease the duration of a crisis. However, there may be a risk of rebound attack after therapy is discontinued.

Also steroids can accelerate avascular necrosis and increase the risk of infection. Thus, their overall role in the acute setting is unclear.

*Sedatives and anxiolytics* are commonly used and show benefit, but should not be used as an alternative to analgesia.

*Spirometry and physiotherapy* are essential in the management of chest crisis.

*Non-pharmacological treatment* includes heat or ice packs, transcutaneous electrical nerve stimulation (TENS), relaxation, acupuncture, music, and massage. The evidence for their efficacy is limited.

*Complementary and alternative* medicine including antioxidants, vitamins, herbal products, glucosamine, magnesium, and zinc are used by some patients but with minimal evidence base.

### 14.1.6 **Progress of the crisis**

Pain seems to be most severe by day 3 of a crisis and starts to decrease by day 6 or 7. The average length of hospital stay seems to be between 9 and 11 days.

Unfortunately, about 10–15% of patients are readmitted to hospital with a painful crisis within 1 week of discharge. This may be due to a hypercoagulable state in the resolving phase leading to recurrence of the crisis but may also be due to premature hospital discharge or the development of withdrawal syndrome after discharge. Therefore, early discharge must be avoided and careful discharge instructions be given to avoid withdrawal outside hospital.

### 14.1.7 **Prevention of painful sickle crises**

Exchange or blood transfusion programs may modify the natural history of the disease and can be used in those with recurrent painful episodes or those thought to be at risk to reduce further crises.

Hydroxyurea decreases the frequency of acute crises, life-threatening complications, and transfusion requirements by increasing foetal Hb levels as well as other postulated mechanisms.

### 14.1.8 **Transition to chronic pain/long-term management**

There are two types of chronic sickle cell pain: chronic pain due to obvious pathology (leg ulcers, avascular necrosis, chronic osteomyelitis) and chronic pain with no obvious signs except the patient's self-report of pain. The pathophysiology of the latter is not fully understood, but may be due to inadequate treatment of recurrent severe acute painful crises and sensitization of the central nervous system.

Once chronic pain sets in, it is usually independent of vasoocclusion and the percentage of HbS, though it will be superimposed with acute painful crises due to vasoocclusion.

Leg ulcers require the input of wound care specialists. Avascular necrosis requires the involvement of orthopaedics, physical therapy, rehabilitation, and rheumatology.

Inevitably with chronic sickle cell pain, slow-release formulations of opioids (e.g., morphine or oxycodone) or long-acting opioids (e.g., methadone) is required together with quick-release formulations for breakthrough pain.

Long-term effects of SCD include disruption to home, work, or education. There are few studies on their chronic pain management. Nonetheless, multidisciplinary pain management including behavioural and psychological treatment (cognitive behavioural therapy) has been shown to be effective and may be required when managing patients with chronic, frequent painful crises. This can help avoid escalating doses of opioids and improve quality of life.

## 14.2 **Thalassaemias**

### 14.2.1 **Clinical features**

These are inherited disorders with reduced synthesis of one or more of the α- or β-chains of Hb. It may be inherited with HbS leading to a sickling condition.

They can present with painful, massive splenomegaly. This is treated with analgesics in the first instance but in extreme situations, a splenectomy can be performed to relieve pain.

These patients also suffer from bone pain due to bone marrow hyperplasia. Commonly, the sternum is the bone involved resulting in mediastinal chest pain.

14.2.2 **Management**

Start with simple analgesics and escalate to strong opioids as required. This is usually only when there has been coinheritance with HbS. The sickling crises are managed as described earlier.

## 14.3 Haemophilia

### 14.3.1 Clinical features

These are inherited coagulation disorders with deficiency of factor VIII (haemophilia A) or factor IX (haemophilia B) most commonly although other rare deficiencies can also lead to similar problems.

They are associated with spontaneous as well as post-traumatic haemorrhages, the frequency and severity being proportional to the degree of clotting factor deficiency.

Bleeding into joints and muscles (i.e., restricted spaces) is a common cause of acute pain in haemophiliacs. Spontaneous internal bleeding is uncommon.

The commonest joints affected are the weight-bearing joints (ankle, knee, hip) but also elbow and shoulder.

Recurrent haemarthroses can lead to chronic haemophiliac arthropathy.

They may also have pain syndromes associated with HIV/AIDS.

### 14.3.2 Management

#### 14.3.2.1 Analgesia

Ranging from cold packs and bandaging to simple analgesics escalating up to opioids.

The use of NSAIDs theoretically may be detrimental due to their antiplatelet effect. However, ibuprofen has been used to control joint pain in haemophiliacs without any change in platelet function, bleeding time, frequency of joint haemorrhages, or frequency of factor infusions. COX-2 inhibitors may be safer due to the lack of antiplatelet effect though these drugs are not popular amongst haematology clinicians.

Avoid intramuscular injections as they can cause further bleeding.

#### 14.3.2.2 Replacement therapy

This is used to treat bleeding episodes, which can lead to rapid improvement in pain symptoms. Replacement with appropriate coagulation factors most commonly factors VIII and IX but also other coagulation factors. Management should be in conjunction with a haemophilia comprehensive care centre, ideally the centre with which the patient is registered.

Higher dose factor VIII may prevent residual-restricted joint movement after an acute haemarthrosis.

The administration of regular prophylactic coagulation factors for children at weight-bearing age has been shown to reduce the incidence of acute haemarthroses, thus preventing the development of chronic haemophilic arthropathy.

### 14.3.2.3 *Joint aspiration*
Following analgesia and immobilization, if pain control is still inadequate joint aspiration with concomitant appropriate recombinant factor cover may reduce pain and improve joint function.

### 14.3.2.4 *Physiotherapy*
Early physiotherapy can prevent the development of chronic haemophilic arthropathy following haemarthrosis.

### 14.3.2.5 *Orthopaedics*
Patients with chronic haemophilic arthropathy may require procedures such as arthrodesis.

### 14.3.2.6 *Steroids*
Painful acute non-infective synovitis complicating acute haemarthrosis can be treated with steroids.

### 14.3.3 **Long-term management**
Recurrent acute pain can have an adverse effect on mood and quality of life in these patients. Therefore, a biopsychosocial assessment with multidisciplinary pain management should be considered.

## 14.4 Lymphoma and other haematological cancers

Lymphoma or lymphoid deposits can cause neuralgic pain. Management involves treating the underlying disorder as well as neuropathic agents such as gabapentin and/or amitriptyline.

### 14.4.1 **Mucositis**
#### 14.4.1.1 *Clinical features*
Mucositis is acute ulceration and inflammation of the oral mucosa. This can be caused by radiotherapy or chemotherapy drugs such as melphalan and methotrexate. The pain can be severe and debilitating.

#### 14.4.1.2 *Management*
*Topical agents* such as EMLA cream and 5% lidocaine can provide good analgesia.

Other solutions used include benzydamine (Difflam®), lidocaine, chlorhexidine (Corsodyl®), soluble paracetamol, sucralfate, salt and soda water, bicarbonate, vitamin E, immunoglobulin, and human placental extract. Topical ketamine rinse has been shown to provide analgesia in severe mucositis for some patients.

In severe mucositis, some of these solutions may be too abrasive and painful (chlorhexidine, benzydamine). The mouthwash can be diluted down with an equal volume of water or sterile saline.

*Parenteral opioids*: PCA or continuous infusion is effective in more severe cases. Transdermal opioids have also been used.

### 14.4.2 **GCSF-induced bone pain**

Granulocyte colony-stimulating factor (GCSF) is used to stimulate the bone marrow and increase the neutrophil count in neutropenic patients. It is also used to stimulate the bone marrow of donor patients before bone marrow harvest. This bone marrow stimulation can induce bone pain. It seems to best respond to simple analgesics rather than opioids.

### 14.4.3 **Generalized pain**

As with many cancer patients, as the disease of the haematology–oncology patient progresses, there is a propensity to suffer from general myalgic and arthralgic pain. These should be treated symptomatically.

## 14.5 **Myeloma**

### 14.5.1 **Clinical features**

This is a neoplastic disease with the proliferation of plasma cells in the bone marrow. It results in bone marrow suppression, lytic bone lesions due to increased osteoclast activity, and the production of monoclonal immunoglobulin paraproteins.

Pain can occur due to

- Myeloma bone pain
- Pathological fractures
- Nerve impingement pain following extramedullary spread (e.g., soft tissue)
- Nerve impingement pain following pathological fracture (including spinal cord compression, nerve root, or peripheral nerve compression).

### 14.5.2 **Management**

*Chemotherapy* as well as *conventional analgesia* is the first-line treatment for myeloma with a high response rate, both in terms of pain relief and suppression of paraproteins. Agents used include oral melphalan, combination chemotherapy including thalidomide and bortezomib (though both can lead to neuropathies), as well as cyclophosphamide and dexamethasone.

*Radiotherapy* is used specifically to treat bone pain of myeloma.

*Bisphosphonates* (sodium clodronate, disodium pamidronate, zoledronic acid) are also used to treat bone pain when conventional analgesics have failed. Mode of action is through the inhibition of osteoclasts.

*Neuropathic agents* such as gabapentin or amitriptyline are used if there is nerve impingement following soft tissue spread or pathological fractures.

*Pathological fractures*: Conventional analgesics, orthopaedic referral, kyphoplasty.

*Spinal cord compression* is a neurosurgical emergency.

## 14.6 Pethidine

It is generally accepted that the use of pethidine (meperidine) is to be discouraged. In particular, the chronic intramuscular use of this opioid should be avoided.

Unfortunately, a significant number of patients with haematological disorders associated with chronic pain (SCD, haemophilia) have had their pain managed with long-term intramuscular pethidine.

In addition, muscle damage and the infection risk with repeated intramuscular injections, its metabolite (norpethidine) is a cerebral irritant and can cause convulsions. The risk of convulsion is further increased by the accumulation of norpethidine as it is excreted by the kidneys, an organ whose function can be impaired in SCD.

Furthermore, these patients have a higher tendency towards addictive behaviour with rapidly escalating pethidine doses despite little improvement in analgesic quality. Attempts at use of alternative opioids can be a source of conflict with these patients and they can be very difficult to manage both in primary care and hospital settings.

Nonetheless, rotation to alternative opioids given by the oral or intravenous route should be sought, as well as the use of analgesic adjuncts. Patient education regarding the harmful effect of chronic intramuscular pethidine should help in their management. Therefore, pethidine should only be used in exceptional circumstances.

## References

Ballas SK (2007). Current issues in sickle cell pain and its management. *Hematology*, **2007**, 97–105.

Benjamin LJ, Dampier CD, Jacox A, *et al.* (1999). Guidelines for the management of acute and chronic pain in sickle cell disease. American Pain Society Practice Guidelines Series, No. 1. American Pain Society, Glenview, IL. Available at www.ampainsoc.org.

Conti C, Tso E, and Browne B (1996). Oral morphine protocol for sickle cell crisis pain. *Maryland Medical Journal*, **45**, 33–5.

Dunlop J and Bennett KC (2006). Pain management for acute sickle cell disease. *Cochrane Database of Systematic Reviews*, **2**, CD003350.

Friedman EW, Webber AB, Osborn HH, and Schwartz S (1986). Oral analgesia for treatment of painful crisis in sickle cell anaemia. *Annals of Emergency Medicine*, **15**, 787–91.

Hurtig AL, Koepke D, and Park KB (1989). Relation between severity of chronic illness and adjustment in children and adolescents with sickle cell disease *Journal of Pediatric Psychology*, **14**, 117–32.

Rees D (2003). Guidelines for the management of acute painful crisis in sickle cell disease. *British Journal of Haematology*, **120**, 744–52.

Robieux IC, Kellner JD, Coppes MJ, *et al.* (1992). Analgesia in children with sickle cell crisis: comparison of intermittent opioids vs continuous intravenous infusion of morphine and placebo controlled study of oxygen inhalation. *Journal of Pediatric Hematology/Oncology*, **9**, 317–26.

Zipursky A, Robieux IC, Brown EJ, *et al.* (1992). Oxygen therapy in sickle cell disease. *American Journal of Pediatric Hematology Oncology*, **14**, 222–8.

# Chapter 15

# Acute pain in patients with renal or hepatic impairment

Ramini Moonesinghe and Sue Mallett

## Key points

- The metabolism and excretion of many analgesic drugs will be altered in the presence of renal or hepatic impairment.
- Some analgesic drugs can cause renal or hepatic damage.
- Protein binding of drugs may be altered by hepatic reduction in production or uraemic displacement from binding sites.
- In renal disease, paracetamol is the simple analgesic of choice.
- Morphine can be used with care in mild to moderate renal disease, but fentanyl or oxycodone may be better alternatives.
- Non-steroidal anti-inflammatory drugs should be avoided in renal disease.
- In hepatic disease with significant impairment, doses of morphine must be reduced and the dosage interval lengthened.
- Fentanyl should be avoided in severe hepatic disease.

## 15.1 Introduction

Acute pain patients with hepatic or renal impairment present an interesting problem to the physician, owing to the impact that liver and kidney dysfunction may have on the metabolism and excretion of analgesic agents and their metabolites. Furthermore, some analgesic agents may aggravate or accelerate existing renal or hepatic disease.

## 15.2 **Pathophysiology of renal impairment**

### 15.2.1 **Renal excretion of drugs**

Renal excretion of drugs and their metabolites in the urine depends on three processes: glomerular filtration, active tubular secretion, and passive tubular reabsorption. How much of a drug enters the tubular filtrate depends on its fractional plasma protein binding and the glomerular filtration rate (GFR). Therefore, a reduction in the GFR will significantly affect renal excretion. Many drug metabolites are in the form of glucuronides, these molecules are excreted by active secretion in the proximal tubule, along carrier mechanisms used for the excretion of uric acid. Analgesic drugs and their metabolites are not subject to reabsorption in the distal tubules.

A GFR of greater than 100mL/min is considered normal. It is now common for estimated GFR to be given as part of the results from the estimation of urea and electrolytes. These figures are sufficiently accurate to guide prescribing of analgesics where renal impairment is mild. Formal creatinine clearance determined that GFR will be available when renal disease is advanced. GFR falls with age, which may compound renal failure from other causes. Kidney disease is classified into five stages as shown in Table 15.1. The level of GFR defines these stages. Where alternative routes of clearance are available, they will be used to greater extent when renal impairment develops.

Predictable adverse effects from analgesic agents may occur in renal disease, owing to the retention of the parent drug and its metabolites: reduced clearance leads to prolonged effect and increased toxicity. The degree of renal impairment, as demonstrated by an estimation of GFR, will influence decisions over analgesic choice. In patients with moderate or mild renal impairment, for example, it may be possible to use reduced doses of morphine; however, this should be avoided altogether in patients with severe renal impairment.

Changes in drug protein binding may occur in uraemic patients. Acidic drugs such as NSAIDs will have reduced plasma protein binding

| Table 15.1 **Renal disease** | | |
|---|---|---|
| **Stage** | **Description** | **GFR** |
| 'At risk' | Risk factors such as diabetes, hypertension, family history, or ethnic group but normal GFR | +90 |
| Stage 1 | Proteinuria | +90 |
| Stage 2 | Proteinuria and mild reduction in GFR | 60–89 |
| Stage 3 | Proteinuria and moderate decrease in GFR | 30–59 |
| Stage 4 | Proteinuria and severe decrease in GFR | 15–29 |
| Stage 5 | Renal failure | <15 |

and therefore an increase in the plasma levels of the unbound 'active' fraction. Basic drugs such as morphine may also be less protein bound, although this is less predictable.

Metabolites of opioid analgesics will accumulate in renal failure; this effect is particularly pronounced with morphine metabolites, which are active and may cause adverse effects. Fentanyl and oxycodone metabolites, however, are inactive, and so these drugs are preferred in patients with renal impairment.

## 15.3 Analgesics in renal impairment

### 15.3.1 Simple analgesics

#### 15.3.1.1 *Paracetamol*

Paracetamol is the simple analgesic of choice in patients with renal impairment.

The risk of developing or worsening renal failure with the use of paracetamol as compared to non-steroidal anti-inflammatory drugs (NSAIDs) is minimal. It has been implicated in the development of analgesic nephropathy, but this is a rare occurrence.

It is metabolized by the liver and may accumulate in uraemic patients due to alterations in hepatic blood flow; furthermore, small studies have shown that its sulphate and glucoronidate metabolites may also accumulate. However, this is unlikely to be of clinical significance if doses of less than 80mg/kg/day are used.

### 15.3.2 **Non-steroidal anti-inflammatory drugs**

NSAIDs should be avoided in patients with any evidence of renal impairment.

NSAIDs are known to cause renal impairment by reducing the production of renal prostaglandin, leading to reduced afferent arteriolar vasoconstriction and thus lowering GFR.

However, NSAID-induced renal dysfunction is generally acute, reversible upon cessation of the agent, and associated with co-morbidities such as hypovolaemia, hypotension, or pre-existing liver or renal disease.

The risk of developing renal impairment with no pre-existing renal disease is very low in acute use of the drugs, but idiosyncratic reactions do occur, particularly interstitial nephritis, which may lead to End-Stage Renal Failure. There is no evidence that differentiates between different NSAIDs in terms of risk of developing renal impairment.

### 15.3.3 Opioids

#### 15.3.3.1 *Codeine/dihydrocodeine*

Codeine is not recommended for use in patients with renal impairment. Codeine is metabolized by cytochrome enzyme P450 to morphine.

Renal disease may cause the accumulation of both the parent drug and its metabolites, all of which are renally excreted. This effect may be seen over several days, where progressive sedation may occur. Although all opioids may cause central nervous system toxicity in overdose, codeine appears to have toxic side effects even when taken at slightly greater than the recommended maximum daily dose. It has also been shown to cause prolonged sedation in patients with dialysis-dependent renal failure.

#### 15.3.3.2 *Morphine*

Morphine should be avoided in patients with significant renal disease. It may be considered in patients with mild or moderate renal impairment, in reduced dosage with increased dose interval; however, other opioid analgesics such as oxycodone or fentanyl should be used in preference.

Morphine is broken down in the liver into two main metabolites: morphine-3-glucuronide (M3G) and morphine-6-glucuronide (M6G). The excretion of both these metabolites, particularly M6G, is renally dependent.

M6G shares many effects and side effects with its parent compound, and as such, its accumulation may cause prolongation of the general effects of morphine. The effects of M6G vary considerably between individuals, with the most potentially harmful problem being delayed sedation; there are several case reports of this occurring in renal failure patients in the literature, usually in association with the administration of high initial loading doses. In this situation, which commonly occurs in post-operative patients who have received high loading doses of morphine in theatre, an alternative maintenance analgesic agent such as fentanyl or oxycodone should be considered.

Although M3G is thought to cause paradoxically heightened pain perception and irritability, these problems are not thought to occur with increased frequency in patients with renal failure. However, M3G may reduce seizure threshold and so morphine should be avoided in patients with renal failure and a history of epilepsy or other seizure activity.

There is potential for serious harm when converting patients from parenteral to oral morphine on the ward. Normally, the equivalent oral dose of morphine would be greater than the parenteral dose; however, the accumulation of metabolites will thus also increase. In this situation, therefore, either the oral equivalent dose should be reduced by one-third or an alternative oral agent with inactive metabolites should be used.

Morphine and its metabolites are effectively cleared by haemodialysis and haemofiltration, but not by continuous ambulatory peritoneal dialysis.

In summary, as a general rule, morphine may be considered safe for use in patients with renal impairment, as long as a large loading dose has not been used and the patient has no history of seizure activity. However, when converting to oral morphine, equivalent dose reduction should be considered to prevent the accumulation of potentially harmful metabolites.

### 15.3.3.3 *Oxycodone*

Oxycodone is the opioid analgesic of choice in patients with renal disease.

Despite the fact that oxycodone is predominantly eliminated via the hepatic route, one study found that its half-life is significantly prolonged in uraemic patients undergoing renal transplantation. However, when compared with morphine, there is less potential for adverse effects, as its metabolites are inactive. It is recommended that if used in renal impairment, oxycodone be cautiously titrated to effect. An example of a suitable 'patient-controlled analgesia (PCA)' regimen would be bolus doses of 1mg oxycodone with a 10min lockout.

### 15.3.3.4 *Fentanyl*

Fentanyl is the second choice synthetic opioid analgesic in renal impairment.

Fentanyl clearance may be reduced in acute renal impairment as it has a high hepatic extraction ratio, and in the presence of uraemia, hepatic blood flow will be altered. However, it has no active metabolites, and clearance has not been shown to be affected by chronic renal failure; thus, it may be used in patients with renal impairment, as long as dose reduction is applied where required in patients with acute uraemia. Fentanyl also is suitable for use in PCA.

### 15.3.3.5 *Tramadol*

Tramadol may be used in patients with renal impairment, with an increased dose interval.

Tramadol is a cyclohexanol derivative that acts on serotoninergic, noradrenergic, and opioid receptors.

Although tramadol is metabolized in the liver, its excretion and that of its metabolites is renally dependent. However, neither tramadol nor its metabolite is known to be nephrotoxic in patients with normal renal function. An increased dosing interval (to 12hr) is recommended for patients with renal impairment; careful observation should be made for possible adverse effects such as myoclonus or hyperreflexia. It should be avoided altogether in patients with a GFR less than 10mL/min (Table 15.2).

**Table 15.2 Summary of the use of analgesic drugs in renal failure**

| Drugs | Comments |
|---|---|
| Alfentanil<br>Fentanyl<br>Ketamine<br>Paracetamol | No significant active metabolites can be used in renal failure |
| Oxycodone | Weakly active metabolite oxymorphone can be used in renal failure |
| Clonidine<br>Gabapentin<br>Hydromorphone<br>Methadone<br>Morphine<br>Tramadol<br>Codeine | Parent drug or active metabolite will accumulate in renal failure, dose size and interval needs to be modified according to the severity of the renal disease |
| NSAIDs<br>Pethidine<br>Codeine | Significant toxicity, accumulation of toxic metabolites to be not recommended in renal failure |

## 15.4 Analgesia in hepatic impairment

### 15.4.1 Pathophysiology of hepatic disease

The liver has a large margin of safety in terms of its biochemical capabilities, and it can also regenerate hepatocytes. Significant hepatocellular damage must occur before clinical manifestations of hepatic disease, such as jaundice, occur. As liver damage occurs, the damaged hepatocytes spill enzymes into the circulation and are detected by liver function tests (LFTs). Alterations in LFTs do not directly reflect metabolic and synthetic function, and are a very crude indicator of the state of liver function, and should always be considered along side the clinical condition of the patient. Serial deterioration of LFTs is a matter for concern, may be a result of other disease processes, such as congestive cardiac failure, poisoning, or malignancy, but does not always reflect alterations in drug handling by the liver.

It is, therefore, more difficult to stage liver disease in terms of its effects on drug metabolism than with renal disease and drug clearance. A general outline is given in Table 15.3.

Adverse effects resulting from the use of analgesic drugs in patients with liver disease may arise via a number of mechanisms, such as alteration in protein binding of drugs, alteration in hepatic blood flow and first pass metabolism, and reduction in hepatic clearance. Drugs that are cleared efficiently by the liver, with high extraction ratios in

| Table 15.3 Liver disease | |
|---|---|
| Stage | Investigations |
| Mild hepatic impairment | Raised AST and ALT |
| Moderate hepatic impairment | Raised AST, ALT, and alkaline phosphatases |
| Severe liver disease | Above, plus raised serum bilirubin, prolonged INR, and reduced albumin |

the normal liver, are more subject to effects on hepatic blood flow, morphine falls into this group. This may be seen in post-operative patients, where the alterations in cardiac output and changes in regional blood flow that accompany general anaesthesia affect liver blood flow. This effect will be particularly pronounced in patients with pre-existing liver disease.

Moderate to severe liver disease may markedly increase the bioavailability of orally administered drugs with high hepatic first pass metabolism.

Obstructive liver disease, due to cholistasis or tumour, will tend to reduce drug clearance of drugs, owing to reduced elimination of the parent drug and its metabolites in the bile. Thus, analgesics may tend to have a longer duration of action and their metabolites will persist for longer than usual.

In cirrhotic liver disease, reduction in plasma protein binding will result in an increase in the 'unbound' and thus 'active' form of a drug, therefore causing increased target effects and necessitating a lower dosage to achieve a desired clinical effect.

### 15.4.2 Simple analgesics

#### 15.4.2.1 *Paracetamol*

In general, paracetamol may be used safely in patients with mild or moderate liver impairment, with the obvious exception of patients with liver failure due to paracetamol overdose.

Paracetamol overdose is a well-known cause of hepatic toxicity, which in its most severe form may progress to acute fulminant liver failure. Cirrhotic patients will have impaired clearance of paracetamol, so potentially increasing the risk of toxicity, especially with the concomitant use of liver enzyme inducing agents such as barbiturates, phenytoin, and alcohol. Therefore, in cirrhotics, paracetamol should be administered in a reduced dose, with appropriate monitoring of hepatic enzymes; however, in patients with severe liver failure, it is best avoided altogether.

### 15.4.2.2 *Non-steroidal anti-inflammatory agents*

NSAIDs may be used in patients with mild or moderate hepatic dysfunction, but the increased bleeding risk owing to platelet inhibition should be considered.

NSAIDs may be associated with elevated liver enzymes in up to 15% of patients, and the NSAID should be stopped if this occurs. No studies are available looking at the effect of NSAIDs in patients with severe hepatic impairment. If using NSAIDs in patients with hepatic disease, liver enzymes should be monitored regularly and treatment stopped if they begin to rise. NSAIDs should not be administered to patients with coagulation disorders or with increased bleeding risk such as from varices or gastric irritation/peptic ulcer disease.

### 15.4.3 **Opioids**

#### 15.4.3.1 *Codeine/dihydrocodeine*

Codeine and its derivative agents should not be used in patients with liver disease.

Codeine itself has a poor affinity for opiate receptors, its analgesic effect is dependent on its hepatic metabolism to morphine (approximately 10% of the administered dose). The remaining 90% is metabolized by the liver to norcodeine and codeine-6-glucuronide, neither of which is significantly active, and are excreted by the kidneys. Thus, impairment of either renal or hepatic function may cause the accumulation of codeine or its metabolites and its use is not recommended.

#### 15.4.3.2 *Morphine*

Morphine may be used with caution in patients with mild or moderate liver impairment, but in reduced dose with increased dose interval. The liver has a large reserve for glucuronidation and there is little evidence of accumulation in mild and moderate disease.

No studies have been conducted looking at morphine usage in patients with severe liver impairment. However, predictable potentially harmful effects may include poor clearance with its sequelae, increased bioavailability, and thus potential for overdosage, as a result of impaired first pass metabolism, and precipitation of hepatic encephalopathy. As a result of this, an initial increase in dose interval, with careful titration of morphine dosage and frequency to effect is to be recommended.

#### 15.4.3.3 *Oxycodone*

Oxycodone may be used with caution in patients with mild or moderate liver impairment, but in reduced dose with increased dose interval.

Oxycodone is metabolized to noroxycodone and oxymorphone by the liver, and these metabolites do have some analgesic and other effects. However, no studies have been conducted specifically looking at the oxycodone use in patients with hepatic impairment. Alterations in hepatic blood flow will lead to impaired clearance. An increase in dosing interval and careful observation for side effects is recommended.

### 15.4.3.4 *Fentanyl*

Dose reduction is required, as fentanyl clearance is likely to be compromised in hepatic impairment.

### 15.4.3.5 *Tramadol*

Tramadol may be used with an increased dosing interval in patients with mild or moderate hepatic impairment (Table 15.4).

Tramadol is broken down in the liver to a number of metabolites including the pharmacologically active *O*-desmethyltramadol.

It should be used with an increased dosage interval, with careful observation for signs of serotoninergic syndrome, such as hyperreflexia and clonus.

| Table 15.4 Summary of the use of analgesic drugs in hepatic impairment | |
| --- | --- |
| **Drug** | **Comments** |
| Alfentanil<br>Fentanyl | Limited data suggest no accumulation in liver impairment |
| Morphine | Liver has large reserve for glucuronidation, reduced doses safe in all but most severe impairment |
| Tramadol | Dose adjustment required, reduced oxidation leads to reduced clearance |
| Amine local anaesthetics | Reduced clearance may lead to toxicity |
| Pethidine | Not recommended for use in liver impairment<br><br>In liver impairment, titrate all analgesics to ensure safety |

## References

The British Medical Association and the Royal Pharmaceutical Society of Great Britain (2008). *BNF* 56th edition. BMJ Publishing Group, London.

Calvey TN and Williams NE, eds. (2001). *Principles and Practice of Pharmacology for Anaesthetists*, 4th edn. Blackwell Science, Oxford.

Davies G, Kingswood C, and Street M (1996). Pharmacokinetics of opioids in renal dysfunction. *Clinical Pharmacokinetics*, **31**, 410–22.

Mercadante S and Arcuri E (2004). Opioids and renal function. *Journal of Pain*, **5**, 2–19.

Merry A and Power I (1995). Perioperative NSAIDS; towards greater safety. *Pain Reviews*, **2**, 268–91.

Murphy EJ (2005). Acute pain management pharmacology for the patient with concurrent renal or hepatic disease. *Anaesthesia & Intensive Care*, **33**, 311–22.

Tegeder I, Lötsch J, and Geisslinger G (1999). Pharmacokinetics of opioids in liver disease. *Clinical Pharmacokinetics*, **37**, 17–40.

# Chapter 16

# Acute pain in the neurological patient

Sam Chong and J. Ganesalingham

> **Key points**
>
> - Acute pain is a common presenting symptom in patients with neurological conditions.
> - Acute onset headache may indicate a life-threatening underlying condition.
> - Lumbosacral and cervical spine pain are commonly caused by degenerative disease but there are sometimes clues to indicate alternative pathologies.
> - Acute pain arising from the peripheral nervous system and muscles are usually inflammatory in origin.
> - A careful history and examination is crucial to assess patients with neurological pain.
> - Opioids may be used in combination of an anti-epileptic or antidepressant drug in the treatment of acute neuropathic pain.

## 16.1 Introduction

Acute pain is a common presenting symptom in patients with neurological conditions. Head and face pain is especially prevalent and acute pain may also affect other parts of the neural axis. Spine pain is common and indeed the lumbosacral and cervical spine are common sites of acute and chronic pain.

The meninges and perineurium are heavily innervated by sensory nerve fibres and are sensitive to a large variety of stimuli, especially mechanical and inflammatory changes. Many forms of acute pain arising from neurological conditions are a form of visceral pain that is difficult to localize. For example, pain radiating from behind the eyes commonly arises from meningeal irritation in the middle cranial fossa and does not necessarily imply pathology in the retro-orbital space. Acute compression of the median nerve at the wrist from a fracture or haematoma often cause pain radiating up the forearm as well as

ALL fingers in the hand. Pain may not be confined to the index, middle, and half of the ring finger, which are innervated by the median nerve.

Back and neck pain is complex and can arise from a number of possible sources. The intervertebral discs themselves, especially the annulus, have a dense nerve supply similar to the longitudinal ligaments in the spine. The facet joints are also heavily innervated. These three structures have a dense supply of sensory and autonomic nerve fibres. Any injuries, causing damage to structures of the spine, can result in further inflammatory pain. For example, the extruded nucleus pulposus from a split intervertebral disc has been shown to cause chemical inflammation of the meninges and perineurium around spinal roots and nerves. Secondary inflammatory pain is also initiated after tissue damage as a part of primary sensitization. Another important component of back pain is reflex paraspinal muscle spasms. This may be a major component in the development of chronic back pain. Experiments performed by Kellgren nearly a century ago have clearly shown that nociceptive pain from back muscles radiate down the leg and can be easily confused with irritation of the sciatic nerve (Kellgren 1938).

## 16.2 Spinal pain: atypical forms

The cervical and lumbosacral spinal segments are mobile, making them more susceptible to degenerative changes. The thoracic vertebrae are splinted by ribs and are relatively fixed. Therefore, pain in this area should not be easily dismissed as just degenerative spinal disease. Many diverse conditions from dissection of the aorta, non-Hodgkin's lymphoma to spinal tuberculosis may present with thoracic spinal pain. Similarly, most degenerative spinal disease is alleviated by rest and made worse by activity. Pain exacerbated by lying down may be caused by a spinal mass as recumbency increases intraspinal pressure.

The practical rule is that acute onset spinal pain needs to be investigated in patients with unexpected neurological symptoms, abnormal signs, systemic illness, or who have a history of past malignancy or chronic infection, especially with the human immunodeficiency virus (HIV). Serious pathology in the spine is rare and the majority of patients with spinal and back pain are caused by degenerative musculoskeletal disease.

## 16.3 Peripheral pain syndromes

Numerous acute pain syndromes arising from the peripheral nervous system are also seen in neurology practice. The most common forms of painful neuropathy in developed countries are caused by metabolic disorders, diabetes, and alcoholism with polyvitamin deficiencies.

These neuropathies tend to be of gradual onset. All forms of neuropathy, however, may be complicated by secondary inflammation and these tend to present with an acute or subacute onset of pain with sensory and motor deficiency.

Diabetic amyotrophy, for example, is a painful acute inflammatory plexopathy with rapid wasting and weakness especially of the quadriceps muscle. Diabetic radiculopathy is less well known. Patients often present with subacute onset pain with numbness in the trunk. Where the lower thoracic roots are affected, they may have focal weakness of the abdominal muscles.

Vasculitic neuropathies can also lead to acute onset pain with motor or sensory deficits. The pattern is common to that of multiple mononeuropathies rather than a symmetrical painful polyneuropathy. Vasculitic neuropathies can either be primary (Churg–Strauss, Wegener's granulomatosis, polyarteritis nodosa, microscopic polyangiitis) or secondary to systemic vasculitis (systemic lupus erythematosus, rheumatoid arthritis, Sjogren's syndrome, sarcoidosis). Fever and pain from other tissues (muscle, eyes, skin, joint) are common in all forms of vasculitic neuropathies and these may sometimes overshadow the painful neuropathy.

Infectious (hepatitis C, HIV, varicella zoster, Lyme disease) or parainfectious neuropathies (Guillain–Barré syndrome or GBS) also present with acute or subacute pain. Back and neck pain caused by inflammation of spinal roots is especially common in patients with GBS and one study had reported that nearly half of all patients report pain greater than 7/10 on the visual analogue scale. This is particularly debilitating in patients with marked weakness who are unable to move their body to get comfortable. Recrudescence of the varicella zoster virus typically causes acute onset pain with delayed development of the rash and vesicles. This can lead on to postherpetic neuralgia (PHN).

Neoplastic (direct infiltration into nervous tissue) or a paraneoplastic syndrome may also cause painful peripheral neuropathy. This is often secondary to cancers of the breast, bronchus, and teratomas. Toxic neuropathies can also occur acutely or subacutely. Arsenic and thallium are well known but rare causes. However, numerous prescribed medications, isoniazid, cisplatin, vincristine, and nitrofurantoin, can also cause acute painful neuropathy.

Searching for the underlying cause in patients with painful neuropathy is important for at least two reasons. First, it gives urgency to initiate appropriate treatment to deal with the underlying condition. This halts the disease process and reduces disability. In vasculitic neuropathies, for example, appropriate immunosuppression will stop damage to another nerve and shorten recovery time. Second, painful neuropathy may be symptomatic of an underlying condition, for example, a neoplasm that will allow early treatment.

Treating the underlying condition would logically relieve acute neuropathic pain but this often takes time. Symptomatic relieve using drugs may be necessary. Placebo-controlled studies of patients with acute herpes zoster provide the best evidence for pharmacotherapy of acute neuropathic pain. Apart from being effective in alleviating PHN, amitriptyline has also been reported to reduce the risk of developing this chronic pain syndrome when initiated at the onset of zoster eruption. Other drugs reported to be effective in alleviating PHN include tramadol, oxycodone, gabapentin, pregabalin, and the 5% lidocaine patch. There has also been small placebo-controlled studies reporting the effectiveness of carbamazepine and gabapentin for alleviating pain from GBS. Steroids, however, were reported not to be effective.

The most recent guidelines have recommended the use of opioids for rapid relief of acute neuropathic pain but in combination with the above mentioned drugs. Careful balance between side effects and efficacy is crucial in selecting the most appropriate drugs for these patients who may be very ill (see Table 16.1).

| Table 16.1 **Management of acute neuropathic pain** (modified from Dworkin et al. 2007) |
| --- |
| **Assessment** |
| • Establish cause and treat appropriately |
| • Measure pain severity |
| • Identify co-morbidities |
| • Explain cause and realistic expectations of pain control |
| **Treatment** |
| • Non-pharmacological measures including the use of splints, supports, regular physiotherapy, TENS |
| • Start pharmacotherapy with either an antidepressant drug (amitriptyline, imipramine, duloxetine) or gabapentinoid (gabapentin or pregabalin) |
| • Topical lidocaine patch for localized pain |
| • Tramadol or oxycodone where there is a breakthrough pain or where pain is severe at onset |
| **Review** |
| • Continue with chosen medications where pain relieve is adequate and tail off opioid (if used) |
| • Use a combination of antidepressant and anti-epileptic drug together with opioid if necessary where there is some but inadequate pain relieve |
| • Withdraw the first drug and change to another of the same or a different group if there is no relieve at all. Combine these changes with a higher dose or a different opioid where appropriate |

Inflammatory muscle diseases such as polymyositis and dermato-myositis may also cause acute pain. Some forms of toxic and congenital myopathies can also be painful. For example, patients with inborn errors of muscle metabolism involving glycogen metabolism may present with muscle pain after exercise. In all cases, the associated rapid muscle destruction may lead to pigmenturia due to myoglobinuria. Identifying and treating the underlying cause is the most effective way of alleviating pain from muscle disease.

## 16.4 Acute head and face pain

Head and face pain is especially prevalent and the causes may be divided into primary headache syndromes or those symptomatic of an underlying pathology some diagnostic entities can be classified as both primary and secondary syndromes. For example, although migraine is usually a primary condition, it may be symptomatic of an underlying syndrome such as mitochondrial cytopathy. Trigeminal neuralgia may be associated with a blood vessel impinging on the nerve, a plaque of multiple sclerosis around the trigeminal root entry zone, or no obvious structural cause. Tables 16.2 and 16.3 are a list of primary and secondary conditions causing headache and facial pain. These tables are not comprehensive but provide a framework for practical classification. It is beyond the scope of this chapter to describe all the conditions cited in Tables 16.2 and 16.3 but some are discussed to aid practical management.

A comprehensive history and clinical examination is important to identify the underlying cause. Correct diagnosis is vital for treating these conditions because a number of them are only amenable to specific therapies. Pain alleviation on its own without formulating a diagnosis will not work in the long term. Excessive use of analgesic drugs may also lead to the development of medication overuse headache (MOH) (see Tables 16.2 and 16.3).

| Table 16.2 Common primary headache pain syndromes |
| --- |
| • Migraine |
| • Tension-type headache |
| • Trigeminovascular headaches: cluster headache, paroxysmal hemicrania, SUNCT, SUNA |
| • Trigeminal neuralgia |
| • Hypnic headaches |
| • Primary exertional headache |
| • Primary thunderclap headache |
| • New onset daily persistent headache |

## Table 16.3 Secondary headache pain syndromes

| Anatomical structure | Pain syndrome |
|---|---|
| Skin | • Herpes zoster |
| Skull | • Paget's disease<br>• Osteoid Osteoma |
| Sinuses | • Infective: sinusitis—bacterial, fungal<br>• Inflammatory: Wegener's granulomatosis<br>• Infiltrative: nasopharyngeal carcinoma |
| Teeth | • Infective: abscess<br>• Idiopathic: empty socket syndrome |
| Eyes | • Glaucoma<br>• Iritis |
| Blood vessels | • Inflammatory: giant cell arteritis, Takayasu's moyamoya, 1° and 2° cranial arteritis<br>• Dissection: carotid and vertebral arteries<br>• Stroke: arterial and venous thrombosis<br>• Haemorrhages: intracerebral, subarachnoid, subdural, extradural |
| Joints | • Temporomandibular joint (Costen's syndrome) |
| Cranial nerves | • Painful neuropathies: oculomotor, trigeminal, glossopharyngeal |
| Other nerves in head and neck | • Occipital, nasociliary, supraorbital neuralgias |
| Meninges | • Inflammatory: connective tissue disease, chemical, or drugs<br>• Infective: bacteria and non-bacterial meningitis<br>• Infiltrative: neoplastic meningitis |
| CSF space | • High pressure: idiopathic intracranial hypertension, high altitude sickness, hypercapnia, malignant hypertension, severe anaemia, or secondary to space occupying lesion<br>• Low pressure: iatrogenic, sexually related, or spontaneous |
| Referred pain | • Neck: acute cervical disc, spinal haemorrhage<br>• Throat: pharyngeal abscess<br>• Heart: myocardial ischaemia or infarction |

### 16.4.1 Sudden onset headaches

Sudden onset headache is defined as headache going from onset to maximum severity within minutes. A number of these headache syndromes are mentioned in Table 16.4. This symptom may indicate potentially life-threatening pathology. They are treated as emergencies requiring urgent investigation and treatment. Although most patients with sudden onset headaches describe their pain as severe, even the milder forms should be treated in the same manner. Additional information about duration and radiation of pain as well as associated neurological symptoms should be sought, although their absence cannot rule out serious underlying pathology. There are patients where in retrospect, the 'sentinel' bleed was missed because they were perceived to be too 'well' to have sustained an intracranial haemorrhage (Table 16.4).

All patients with sudden onset headache should have an urgent computed tomography (CT) brain scan and if no contraindications, a lumbar puncture to look for evidence of blood or its breakdown products. This is generally sufficient in most patients although CT angiography or even formal intra-arterial digital subtraction angiography (IADSA) should rarely be considered even when CT and cerebrospinal fluid (CSF) examination is normal. Sudden onset headache caused by dissection of the aneurysm vessel wall without bleeding into the subarachnoid space has been reported.

### 16.4.2 Subarachnoid haemorrhage

Subarachnoid haemorrhage from intracranial aneurysms is associated with a high incidence of mortality and morbidity. It is also potentially treatable by neurosurgery or interventional neuroradiology. Therefore, great care is taken to search for the diagnosis before a catastrophic bleed occurs. Studies have reported incidences of between 11% and 40% of patients with sudden onset headache having an eventual diagnosis of subarachnoid haemorrhage. Patients with collagen vascular

---

**Table 16.4 Condition that may present as sudden onset headache**

- Intracerebral, subarachnoid both intracranial and spinal
- Dissection of carotid or vertebral arteries
- Cerebral venous thrombosis
- Acute blockage of CSF pathway
- Pituitary apoplexy

**Primary headache syndromes**
- Exertional
- Sexually related
- Thunderclap

disease (e.g., Ehlers–Danlos, Peutz–Jaeger), long-standing uncontrolled hypertension (renal artery stenosis, polycystic kidney disease, coarctation of the aorta) and where two or more members of the immediate family have intracranial aneurysmal bleeds are at a higher risk of developing intracranial aneurysms.

### 16.4.3 Dissection of carotid or vertebral arteries

Dissection of the carotid and vertebral arteries was thought to be caused by high-velocity deceleration injuries and associated with a high incidence of mortality. It is now known that even minor trauma can cause dissection of one of these neck vessels. The risk of catastrophic intracranial haemorrhage is small and only when dissection of the intracranial portion of the vertebral artery is involved. It is the sudden reduction of blood flow and/or embolization of clots from the damaged vessel wall that is the main risk of ischaemic strokes in these patients. To minimize this, patients are usually anticoagulated although this has not been tested in large placebo-controlled studies. Acute pain in the neck or head before the development of hemiparaesis, ataxia, or cranial nerve palsy should arouse the suspicion of dissection of a neck vessel. A Horner's syndrome contralateral to the affected side caused by damage to the sympathetic chain in the neck may sometimes be seen. Fibromuscular dysplasia of blood vessels is thought to be a risk factor for dissection.

### 16.4.4 Cerebral venous thrombosis

Sudden onset headache with the development of bilateral neurological signs or symptoms should alert clinicians to the possibility of venous sinus thrombosis. Dehydration, treatment with some antineoplastic medications or oestrogen-containing contraceptive pill, and cranial infections (inner ear, orbital cellulitis, sinusitis) are some predisposing factors. These patients should also be screened for procoagulant tendency: factor V Leiden, lupus coagulant, and antithrombin III deficiency. The CT brain scan may show multiple areas of haemorrhage and enhanced scans may show the empty-delta sign where the superior sagittal sinus fails to opacify. Prompt anticoagulation may be life saving although once again, this treatment has never been subjected to large placebo-controlled trials.

### 16.4.5 Acute blockage of CSF pathway

Sudden blockage to CSF can cause acute onset headache, usually with loss of consciousness. This is a true neurosurgical emergency that requires urgent action that may be life-saving. This diagnosis should be suspected in patients known to have intracranial ventricular shunt(s) and congenital malformations such as Arnold–Chiari malformation or skull platybasia. Any sudden change in intracranial posterior fossa pressure such as bleeding or swelling into a space occupying lesion or haemorrhagic transformation of a cerebellar stroke may also cause sudden blockage to the third ventricle or aqueduct of Sylvius. A third ventricular papilloma causing intermittent blockage of the aqueduct is well described but a very rare cause of intermittent sudden headache with episodes of loss of consciousness.

### 16.4.6 **Pituitary apoplexy**

Haemorrhage into a pituitary adenoma can cause sudden onset headache. This condition is more common is younger men and may be misdiagnosed as meningitis or recreational drug abuse. The associated features of visual impairment and oculomotor nerve palsy may help localize the anatomical location of the pathology. Previous case series have reported that the neuroimaging, especially just a CT brain scan alone may be missed if dedicated pituitary views are not performed. Management is conservative in most instances but pituitary decompression may be necessary when vision is affected.

### 16.4.7 **Exertional, sexual activity, and thunderclap headaches (primary sudden onset headaches)**

Headache of sudden onset may precede exertion (exertional headache), sexual arousal (headache associated with sexual activity), or where no cause is found, thunderclap headaches. Studies have reported that up to 75% of patients with this symptom fall into this category of primary sudden onset headache. Some of these conditions overlap as well. Many patients with headache associated with sexual activity may also have exertional headache. In all circumstances, a thorough clinical assessment backed up by appropriate investigations is necessary. Reassurance that the headache, in spite of its severity, is benign and that it may spontaneously remit is usually sufficient for most patients. Where pharmacotherapy is necessary, indometacin appears to have the best evidence based.

## 16.5 **Primary headache syndromes**

Migraine and tension-type headache (TTH) remain the two most common types of primary headache in the population. These two may coexist in the same patient, often together with secondary MOH, giving rise to chronic daily headache (CDH). The recognition of all these diagnostic entities and methods to deal with them are important for the alleviation of CDH.

### 16.5.1 **Migraine**

Migraine is common and relatively easy to diagnose when associated with aura. Excellent reviews of this condition are available in many books and published articles. Management of this condition can be summarized as identifying trigger factors and avoiding them, acute alleviation and long-term prophylaxis. Migraine in young women is associated with an increased risk of ischaemic heart and cerebrovascular disease. Advice on smoking cessation and avoiding the use of oestrogen contraception is necessary.

### 16.5.2 TTH

Tension-type headaches are almost universally experienced but may have different forms: infrequent, frequent, chronic, and with or without pericranial tenderness. Strict delineation from migraine headaches is difficult. The absence of photophobia, phonophobia, and nausea together with the lack of aggravation with exertion make TTH more likely than migraine. Symptom relief of TTH should concentrate on physical methods: massage, hot and cold packs, and acupuncture. Cognitive behaviour therapy and biofeedback training may also help. Where drugs are used, courses of prophylactic therapy is preferable to the regular use of acute pain relieve.

### 16.5.3 Trigeminal autonomic cephalalgias

This group of conditions includes cluster headache (CH), paroxysmal hemicrania (PH), Short-lasting Unilateral Neuralgiform headache with Conjunctival injection and Tearing (SUNCT).

These conditions are relatively rare but important to recognize because some of them are only amenable to specific therapy. CH is the most common and typically affects middle-aged, predominantly men who are heavy smokers. Episodes of severe unilateral pain around the periorbital area lasting 20–60min, associated with tearing and nasal congestion are the usual features. The attacks have a periodicity, occurring commonly at early hours of the morning, and with increased frequency during the summer solstice and winter equinox. Acute attacks respond well to triptans administered either by injection or by inhalation and also to breathing high concentration of oxygen. Prophylactic treatment with verapamil and lithium has been shown to be effective and a short course of oral prednisolone may also terminate a bout. The features of CH in women have been reported to be more migraine-like with nausea and vomiting.

PH may have many of the features of CH. It is, however, more common in women, attack typically lasts between 5 and 20min and responds very well to indometacin. Attacks of SUNCT lasts for even shorter periods of time; typically from seconds up to 4–5min but are frequent, up to 20 or more in a day. The associated features of tearing and conjunctival injection are necessary to make this diagnosis. In these patients, it is important to exclude a structural abnormality around the pituitary. A variety of medications including lamotrigine, gabapentin, and topiramate have been reported to be effective.

## 16.6 **Secondary headache syndromes**

Although relatively rare, the early identification and practical management of these conditions avoid prolonged suffering and potentially serious consequences.

### 16.6.1 **Low pressure headaches**

Headaches caused by low cerebrospinal pressure may be iatrogenic after therapeutic or inadvertent dural puncture, sexually related or 'spontaneous' where a leak from spinal root sheath may sometimes be found. Spontaneous intracranial hypotension has a reported incidence of 5 per 100 000, commonly affecting women in their fourth decade. Associated disorders such as Marfan's, Ehlers–Danlos syndrome type II, autosomal dominant polycystic kidney disease, and neurofibromatosis type 1 have been reported in up to two-third of cases.

This is typically orthostatic headache, gradually worsening over 15min after standing and improving after lying down. The headache is thought to be caused by downward displacement of the brain due to the loss of CSF buoyancy, exerting traction on pain-sensitive structures. Associated symptoms include posterior neck pain or stiffness, photophobia, nausea, and vomiting: symptoms of meningeal irritation. Impaired hearing associated with tinnitus or vertigo from pressure changes via the perilymph or stretching of the vestibulocochlear nerve is also reported. Magnetic resonance imaging (MRI) with gadolinium is the preferred investigation and may show characteristic features including subdural fluid collections, enhancement of pachymeninges, engorgement of venous structures, pituitary hyperemia, and sagging of the brain. Misdiagnosis of this syndrome and attempts at draining the associated subdural collections usually make the problem worse. Conservative management is the mainstay including bed rest, oral rehydration, generous caffeine intake, and the use of an abdominal binder. Steroids, intravenous caffeine, or theophylline have all been advocated but not tested in large placebo-controlled studies. Autologous blood patch may be used if the leak site is identified. The key is to be aware of this condition and request cranial MRI with enhancement in patients with orthostatic headaches.

### 16.6.2 **Giant cell arteritis**

This is a condition exclusively in patients over the age of 50 and is uncommon in those under 65. The pain in giant cell arteritis (GCA) is non-specific, reflecting the diffuse nature of this condition. GCA is also associated with polymyalgia rheumatica, where there may be diffuse muscle pain. Headache in GCA is usually of subacute onset and continuous but may also be acute and intermittent. Jaw claudication and temporal artery tenderness are helpful markers when present. This condition is typically associated with a high erythrocyte sedimentation rate (ESR) but normal levels in biopsy proven cases are well described. Practical management of GCA is to have a high index of suspicion, check ESR, and start high dose steroids early. This avoids the risk of blindness where the ophthalmic artery is involved. An early biopsy of the affected temporal artery, ideally 1cm in length should be sought. The side effects of prolonged steroid therapy are well known and can only be offset by the knowledge of a biopsy proven diagnosis.

## 16.7 **Summary**

Acute pain is commonly seen in neurology practice and may be caused by many conditions. Thorough history and examination to formulate a diagnosis is especially important for this group of patients. Just using analgesics alone for symptom relieve is not appropriate and may exacerbate the underlying condition.

## References

Dubinsky RM, Kabbani H, El-Chami Z, Boutwell C, Ali H; Quality Standards Subcommittee of the American Academy of Neurology. (2004). Practice parameter: treatment of postherpetic neuralgia: an evidence-based report of the Quality Standards Subcommittee of the American Academy of Neurology. *Neurology*, **63**, 959–65.

Dworkin RH, O'Connor AB, Backonja M, *et al.* (2007). Pharmacologic management of neuropathic pain: evidence based recommendations. *Pain*, **132**, 237–51.

Headache Classification Committee of the International Headache Society. (2004). The International Classification of Headache Disorders. *Cephalalgia*, **24**, 9–160.

Hughes RAC, Wijdicks EFM, Barohn R, *et al.* (2005). Supportive care for patients with Guillain-Barré Syndrome. *Archives of Neurology*, **62**, 1194–8.

Kellgren JH (1938). Observations on referred pain arising from muscles. *Clinical Medicine*, **3**, 175–90.

Zakrzewska JM and Harrison S, eds. (2002). *Assessment and Management of Orofacial Pain, Pain Research and Clinical Management*, vol. 14, 1st edn. Elsevier Science, Amsterdam.

# Chapter 17

# Acute pain in chronic opiate users

Brigitta Brandner and Sanjay Bajaj

### Key points

- The main goals in treating perioperative pain are effective analgesia and prevention of withdrawal.
- An acute pain management plan should be formulated and agreed with the patient.
- Discharge planning is only successful if the psychosocial background of the patient is considered.

## 17.1 Introduction

The management of acute pain in opioid-dependent patients can be challenging as it is well recognized that opioid-dependent patients report higher pain scores. Patients with underlying chronic pain often find themselves in a vicious circle resulting in repeated hospital admission and even surgery. Opioid use for non-malignant pain is socially acceptable within the recommendations of the British Pain Society (2004) for the appropriate use of opioids for persistent non-cancer pain; however, patients who have been addicted to opioids and related drugs are exposed to a higher risk of relapse. Addiction to opioids is rare in patients with chronic pain; however, there are currently an estimated 327 000 people addicted to opiate and or crack cocaine in the United Kingdom. The National Institute for Clinical Excellence (NICE) has issued guidelines on maintenance and abstinence therapy, which is an integral part of acute pain treatment.

In severe acute pain, opioid therapy remains a cornerstone, however exploring non-opioid options to treat pain can reduce escalating opioid requirements. Following the World Health Organization (WHO) Pain Ladder, adjuvants such as antidepressants and anti-epileptics may be incorporated depending on the nature of pain. Non-pharmacological option should be encouraged such as TENS, acupuncture, and hypnosis. Psychological support can help to reduce stress and anxiety.

A clear understanding of the differences with regard to physical dependence, tolerance, abuse, addiction, and pseudoaddiction are crucial to set up appropriate treatment plans.

## 17.2 The elements of drug misuse

### 17.2.1 Addiction

Addiction is a compulsive drug-seeking behaviour that results from recurring drug intoxication. Physical dependence and the emergence of withdrawal symptoms were once believed to be the key features of addiction, but craving and relapse can occur weeks and months after withdrawal symptoms are long gone.

### 17.2.2 Physical dependence

Physical dependence may develop within days and is an expected consequence of drug use and is not addiction. It is characterized by the compulsion to take the drug in order to experience its physical effects. On cessation of the drug or administration of an antagonist intense withdrawal symptoms occur. Patients who use opioids for pain relief may be physically dependent on them although few may be psychologically dependent.

### 17.2.3 Tolerance

Tolerance is a progressively decreasing response to repeated dosage of a drug. This has been demonstrated in animals and volunteer studies. It classically occurs with morphine. The adaptive changes can be explained by a right shift of the opioid response curve though progressive loss of receptor site action, functional uncoupling of opioid receptors from GTP subunit decrease agonist-binding affinity and loss of receptors from cell surface. In chronic pain, once a dose has been established tolerance is seldom a problem. Acute opioid tolerance is a new concept described in animal models. It is more likely to occur with large doses of short-acting drugs.

### 17.2.4 Pseudoaddiction

This is described as a drug-seeking behaviour in patients in severe pain and is due to the pharmacokinetics of a short-acting opioid such as pethidine with a short onset and offset of action.

### 17.2.5 Maladaptation

Care needs to be taken once the patient shows loss of control over use, craving, preoccupation despite adequate pain relief, and continued use despite ill effect. Behaviours such as earlier prescription seeking, unsanctioned escalation, requesting specific drugs, various sources, and coexistence of illicit drug use should prompt concern.

### 17.2.6 Cross-tolerance

Tolerance implying an intake of larger doses to obtain the initial effect occurs also with other opioid agonists and is called cross-tolerance. This can also be incomplete, when the initial opioid can be replaced with another one that produces a milder abstinence syndrome.

## 17.3 Opioid rotation

There are numerous reports describing improvement or adverse effects from opioids after switching to an alternative opioid. Switching the opioid 'opioid rotation' allows the metabolites to be eliminated while maintaining analgesia with a strong opioid. This strategy can be particularly useful when the toxicity is severe and/or pain is not well controlled. Switching the opioid requires the use of equianalgesic dose tables. Given the interindividual variability in response to various opioids, these should be viewed as guidelines and close monitoring of patient is essential. There is no sound evidence to suggest superiority of one opioid over another, but some theoretical support of methadone as a useful second-line opioid.

## 17.4 Treatment plan

The main goal for treating acute pain in opioid-dependent patients is satisfactory pain relief, preventing withdrawal, and psychological support. Patients on chronic opioid therapy have often a background of chronic illness or malignancy. It is important to get familiar with the medical background. The general practitioner, palliative care practitioner, or pain management consultant will be able to confirm opioid medication. In dealing with the addicted patient, it is essential to be familiar with common treatments for addiction.

### 17.4.1 Methadone maintenance

Methadone is a synthetic opioid agonist with a long half-life of 12–100hr; it has slow onset and no 'rush'. Opioid tolerance does not eliminate the possibility of methadone overdose, iatrogenic, or otherwise. Deaths have been reported during conversion to methadone from chronic, high-dose treatment with other opioid agonists and during the initiation of methadone treatment of addiction in subjects previously abusing high doses of other agonists. Methadone is an effective analgesic in acute and chronic pain. It is a racemic mixture, which includes an NMDA antagonist and can therefore have an unexpected high potency. Its analgesic effect lasts 4–8hr and a steady-state plateau is reached in days to weeks.

Methadone for maintenance therapy (MMT) is typically dosed between 60 and 120mg/day, fixed or flexible dosing. The success of therapy is dependent on correct dosing and psychosocial support.

### 17.4.2 Buprenorphine

Buprenorphine is a thebaine derivative used for maintenance therapy, usually given by the sublingual route in opiate dependence. It is prescribed 0.8 to 4mg sublingually as a single daily dose. Its analgesic effect is due to partial agonist activity at μ-opioid receptors. An overdose cannot be easily reversed although overdose is unlikely in substance misusers or people with tolerance to opioids. This therapy has a higher relapse rate than high MMT (NICE 2007 Level I). People who are less opioid dependent are more likely to achieve successful abstinence with this therapy. However, for the pain clinician buprenorphine poses a problem due to the unpredictability in its interaction with other opioid therapies and with a elimination half-life of 20–37hr.

### 17.4.3 Naltrexone

Naltrexone, an opioid receptor antagonist, is used for abstinence therapy for alcohol and opioids. When given orally its action is between 24 and 48hr and as a depot injection 3–4 monthly. In the United Kingdom, there is little experience in treating patients on this therapy who require acute pain management. In emergencies such as cases of acute severe pain, higher doses of opioid analgesics may be used with extreme caution to override the blockade produced by naltrexone. The narcotic dose needs to be carefully titrated to achieve adequate pain relief without oversedation or respiratory suppression. If a patient is taken off naltrexone and put on an opioid analgesic, he or she should be abstinent from the narcotic for at least 3–5 days before resuming naltrexone treatment.

### 17.4.4 Providing satisfactory pain relief

Patients can have unrealistic expectation about the outcome of a new treatment or surgery and it is crucial to state that complete pain relief may not be achieved. The patient should be made aware of the nature of their exaggerated pain response and also be informed on the available techniques before surgery, such as in a preassessment clinic. This reduces anxieties and fear and will improve coping. Physiologically, the thermal and nociceptive thresholds are lowered due to central sensitization, the depletion of endogenous opioids with downregulation of secondary messenger systems increases the requirement for opioids.

As pain is one of the most important factors to trigger the stress response it is essential to treat pain promptly. Even after long-term abstinence, the stress response is impaired.

A treatment plan for acute pain in drug-dependent patients guides the health carers involved. Patients are identified as early as possible and are referred to the specialist Acute Pain Team to form an individualized plan, which is discussed with the patient, agreed, and then liaise with all care workers involved. This can be a difficult task in the addicted patient, who is admitted frequently after trauma and infection manifesting in endocarditis and abscesses. Inadvertent intra-arterial injection causing severe ischaemic pain may lead to amputation of the affected limb. Phantom limb pain is not uncommon as preamputation pain is often severe.

Patients who are on maintenance therapy under the care of the drug dependency services or general practitioner have to have their doses confirmed. To prevent withdrawal before dose confirmation, a dose as low as 10mg of methadone is effective; however, positive urine toxicology is mandatory.

### 17.4.5 Assessment

Patients with underlying history of chronic pain or addiction require a thorough assessment after life-threatening conditions have been controlled. The initial consultation in the addicted patient should include physical (human immunodeficiency virus, hepatitis B and C) and mental health such as anxiety, depression, and personality disorders are common. Previous and current records have to be attained. Establishing the social circumstances with current health care providers will facilitate discharge. Particular attention has to be paid to the drug history, and urine toxicology is mandatory in the addicted patient. Current maintenance therapy has to be confirmed with the provider either the general practitioner or the drug dependency unit.

## 17.5 Suitable techniques of pain management

All regular pain medication has to be continued as long as possible orally, as inadvertent discontinuation can lead to severe exacerbation and withdrawal. There is occasionally a misconception that all opioids should be withdrawn before surgery. Clinical experience shows that it is often best to use a single full opioid receptor agonist with little euphoric effect such as morphine. In the addicted patient, drugs, such as codeine, tramadol, oxycodone, pethidine, and diamorphine, that have the potential to be abused are best avoided.

If only the parenteral route is available, then all opioids should be converted into a parenteral dose (Table 17.1) with morphine as the reference drug. Patient-controlled analgesia is a safe method of delivering opioids. Morphine is often first-line opioid used in conjunction with non-opioid medication. Patients who are opioid tolerant require manyfold higher doses and are less likely to suffer from side effects

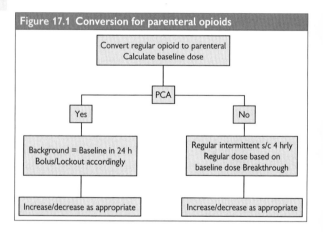

| Table 17.1 Equianalgesic doses | | |
|---|---|---|
| Opioid | Equivalent dose (30 mg codeine) | Potency (vs morphine) |
| Codeine | 30 mg | 1/10 |
| Tramadol | 30 mg | 1/10 |
| Hydrocodone | 5 mg | 0.6 |
| Morphine | 3 mg | 1 |
| Oxycodone | 1.5–2 mg | 1.5–2 |
| Morphine IV/IM | 0.75 mg | 4 |
| Hydromorphone | 0.6 mg | 5 |
| Buprenorphine | 0.075 mg | 40 |
| Fentanyl | 0.03–0.06 mg | 50–100 |

Adapted from http://www.pallcare.unimelb.edu.au/research/documents/
EMRPCCOpioidConversionGuidetoPracticeOctober2008FINAL.pdf

Figure 17.1 Conversion for parenteral opioids

such as respiratory depression. A background infusion can address the underlying requirement with an altered bolus setting. Ultrashort-acting opioids such as remifentanil may lead to acute tolerance and worsen pain in the opioid-dependent patient. The conversion of methadone to morphine can be difficult.

If regional blockade or local anaesthetic limb blocks are used, then the underlying dependency has to be addressed to avoid withdrawal.

As soon as oral intake is possible, the patient should be converted to all oral medication. The discharge planning will be in conjunction with the general practitioner, and possibly in follow-up clinic as an escalation in opioid requirement from preoperative levels is of serious concern.

Some patients will suffer from 'excruciating pain' despite high opioid use. Alternative agents such as sedatives, antipsychotic agents, or NMDA antagonists can be prescribed. The response can be unpredictable and respiratory depression is likely and the patient should transferred to a high dependency unit for monitoring. This structured approach has led to good patient satisfaction and raised the awareness within clinicians involved.

### 17.5.1 Withdrawal

The clinical syndrome is produced by the withdrawal of an opioid drug from a opioid-dependent individual either by cessation of the drug or by the administration of an antagonist, such as naloxone or naltrexone. Initial symptoms and signs may develop immediately after the administration of an opioid antagonist or up to 48hr after cessation or reduction in dosage of the opioid, depending upon the half-life of the drug concerned. These include restlessness, mydriasis, lacrimation, rhinorrhea, sneezing, piloerection, yawning, perspiration, restless sleep, and aggressive behaviour. Severe manifestations include muscle spasms, backaches, abdominal cramps, hot and cold flashes, insomnia, nausea, vomiting, diarrhoea, tachypnoea, hypertension, hypotension, tachycardia, bradycardia, and cardiac dysrhythmias. Seizures may be observed in neonates.

The management of withdrawal in the acute pain setting is mainly pharmacological either with substitution of the drug or with a long-acting opioid such as methadone. Agents such as clonidine and sedatives mitigate symptoms and signs of withdrawal. Withdrawal of longer-acting opioids such as methadone produced a withdrawal syndrome with a more delayed onset, milder severity, and prolonged duration. Withdrawal is rarely fatal.

The withdrawal syndrome produced by the administration of naloxone is intense, occurs within 5min, peaks at approximately 30min, and subsides within 2hr.

### 17.5.2 Conversion to intravenous opioids

It requires clinical experience to convert opioids safely as patients. There is no hard evidence that one opioid is better than another; however some patients seem to tolerate one better than another. Oral opioids need to be converted to parenteral administration according to their bioavailability, that is, 10mg oral morphine equates to 5mg intravenous morphine. Conversion of methadone can be difficult as the morphine:methadone ratio does not correlate linear. Transdermal fentanyl (fentanyl patch) can be converted to parenteral morphine, for example, a 50mcg/hr patch equivalent to oral morphine 100mg in 24hr or 50mg intravenous morphine.

### 17.5.3 **Psychological support**

There is little in the literature on the needed support for this patient group. However, depression and anxiety with a background of uncontrolled pain can be very distressing. Liaison psychiatric input can be very helpful particularly in the 'suicidal' patient. Integrating psychological support into the inpatient setting is rare; however, in paediatric and adolescent ward more common and their use in this situation is to be evaluated.

### 17.5.4 **Planning discharge**

It is essential to establish a therapeutic trustful relationship with the patient in order to address the issue of opioid reduction. However, once the acute pain has settled, the patients are often more motivated to return home. This is dependent on social factors. In complex patients, a multidisciplinary meeting with nurses, medical team, Acute Pain Team, DDU key worker, physiotherapist, occupational therapist, and social worker, occasionally psychiatrist can be useful.

In practice, intravenous opioids are converted to a slow release opioid preparation such as slow release morphine, as this has less euphoric effects. The reduction of the oral opioids is negotiated with the patient according to their pain. The amount of methadone can be increased temporarily for its analgesic effects, this is liaised with the DDU.

## References

Ayonrinde OT and Bridge DT (2000). The rediscovery of methadone for cancer pain management. *Medical Journal of Australia*, **173**, 536–40.

Doverty M, White JM, Somogyi AA, *et al*. (2001). Hyperalgesic responses in methadone maintenance patients. *Pain*, **90**, 91–6.

Jage J and Bey T (2000). Postoperative analgesia in patients with substance abuse disorders Part 1. *Acute Pain*, **3**, 141–156.

Goldstein RZ and Volkow ND (2002). Drug addiction and its underlying neurobiological basis: neuroimaging evidence for the involvement of the frontal cortex. *American Journal of Psychiatry*, **159**, 1642–52.

Guignard B, Bossa AE, Coste C, *et al*. (2000). Acute opioid tolerance: intraoperative remifentanil increases postoperative pain and morphine requirement. *Anesthesiology*, **93**, 409–17.

Rapp SE, Ready LB, and Nessly ML (1995). Acute pain management in patients with prior opioid consumption: a case-controlled retrospective review. *Pain*, **61**, 195–201.

Woodhouse A, Ward ME, Mather LE, *et al*. (1999). Intra subject variability in postoperative patient controlled analgesia (PCA): is the patient equally satisfied with morphine, pethidine and fentanyl? *Pain*, **80**, 545–53.

# Chapter 18

# Acute pain in peripheral vascular disease

Arif H. Ghazi and Obi Agu

> **Key points**
>
> - Pain in vascular disease is often severe.
> - Atherosclerosis is the commonest cause of ischaemic pain.
> - Angioplasty, stents, and surgical revascularization should be attempted to treat the underlying cause.
> - Pain relief is also aimed at neuropathic and sympathetic components of pain.
> - In end stage ischaemic disease, amputation may be necessary often leading to long-term pain.

## 18.1 Introduction

Pain is a common feature of most vascular diseases. Ischaemic pain is caused by an imbalance between tissue oxygen delivery and metabolic demand. This is due to a reduction in blood flow as often the result of vasoconstriction, narrowing, or obstruction by atheroma or embolus, when oxygen supply can no longer keep up with increased demand. Ischaemic pain is characteristic and may be mild to severe. It presents with classical symptoms such as angina due to myocardial ischaemia or claudication and rest pain in lower limb ischaemia.

Peripheral artery occlusive disease can be graded using the Fontaine stages:

- I: mild pain on walking claudication
- II: severe pain on walking relatively shorter distances (intermittent claudication)
- III: pain while resting
- IV: loss of sensation to the lower part of the extremity
- V: tissue loss (gangrene).

Peripheral vascular diseases are classified according to the anatomical structure affected (Table 18.1).

| **Table 18.1 Classification of peripheral vascular disease** |
|---|
| **Medium size arteries** |
| Arteriosclerosis obliterans (ASO) |
| Thromboangiitis obliterans (TAO) |
| Acute arterial occlusion |
| Arterial aneurysm |
| **Other arterial disease** |
| Entrapment syndrome |
| Compartment syndrome |
| **Diseases of small arteries** |
| Embolism |
| Collagen vascular disease |
| Congenital arteriovenous aneurysm |
| Cold injuries (also affect local microcirculation) |
| Pernio syndrome |
| Trench/immersion foot |
| Frostbite |
| **Diseases of microcirculation** |
| Vasospastic disease |
| Raynaud's disease/phenomenon |
| Acrocyanosis |
| Livedo reticularis |
| Vasodilating disease |
| Erythromelagia |
| **Diseases of peripheral veins and lymphatics** |
| Diseases of the veins |
| Acute venous occlusion |
| Thrombophlebitis |
| Deep venous thrombosis |
| Chronic venous disease |
| Post-thrombotic (post-phlebetic) syndrome |
| Varicose veins |
| Disease of the lymphatics |
| Lymphoedema |

## 18.2 **Pathophysiology**

Atherosclerosis is the commonest underlying cause of chronic ischaemia. Plaque development is associated with arterial wall remodelling and increased intima-medial wall thickness reducing the vessel diameter and inflow in response to metabolic demand. The resulting ischaemia reduces the formation of adenosine triphosphate, leading to acidosis and the release of metabolites including lactate, serotonin, histamine, bradykinin, adenosine, and reactive oxygen radicals.

These substances stimulate chemosensitive and mechanoreceptive receptors of unmyelinated nerve cells in the tissue and vessel. The impulses are transmitted via the ascending spinal pathway to the thalamus and cerebral cortex.

## 18.3 Evaluation of patient

### 18.3.1 History

Peripheral vascular disease commonly presents with intermittent claudication, the patient will describe calf, thigh, or buttock pain, which occurs during exercise, particularly walking, but ceases when exercise stops. At early stages of the disease, patients may be able to 'walk through' the pain, but as the disease progresses the patient will have to stop after only a few feet. More severe cases may present with rest pain and tissue loss with ulceration and gangrene with or without claudication. Atherosclerosis is a systemic disease. Patients may, therefore, present with concomitant ischaemic heart, cerebrovascular, and renovascular disease. Older males are more commonly affected.

Risk factors for peripheral vascular disease include

- Age
- Male gender
- Smoking
- Hyperlipidaemia
- Diabetes mellitus
- Family history
- Sedentary lifestyle and obesity

When considering a pain history, onset, localization, distribution, intensity, duration, aggravating, and relieving factors are important.

Intermittent claudication is precipitated by exercise of contracting muscles and relieved by rest. Pain is often localized to the affected muscle group, which may assist with clinical diagnosis of level or location of the disease. The calf is most commonly affected. Although often straightforward, spinal claudication from spinal stenosis may mimic the diagnosis. Rest pain is persistent and worse at night. Pain is described as burning, throbbing, and agonizing. Some relief may be achieved by dangling the foot from the bedside or sleeping in a chair, taking advantage of gravity. Continuous pain may also be produced by sudden arterial occlusion, ulceration, or gangrene, ischaemic neuropathy due to circulatory insufficiency, inflammation of arteries, veins, or lymphatics, and congestion of a limb.

The acutely ischaemic limb is painful, pale, pulseless, and perishing with cold (poikilothermia). Paraesthesia and paralysis are often late and indicative of critical limb-threatening ischaemia (6 Ps).

Inadvertent intra-arterial injection of drugs can also cause severe acute ischaemia, commonly seen in drug misusers but also iatrogenic such as inadvertent injection of irritant injectates such as thiopental.

## 18.4  Management of ischaemic pain

Patients with acute ischaemia are in severe pain requiring frequently strong opioids whilst waiting for invasive treatment. Treatment is aimed at the underlying disease and includes angioplasty, stents, or surgical revascularization if feasible.

Pre-emptive epidural analgesia is indicated in severe pain unresponsive to escalating opioid use; however, anticoagulation in these patients can be a problem for the safe insertion of an epidural catheter.

### 18.4.1  Medical therapy

This strategy is aimed at improving ischaemia.

Where acute occlusion occurs, heparinization and fibrinolytic therapy, for example, urokinase, a tissue plasminogen activator, may have a role. This is of less value in chronic occlusions.

Vasodilators can be helpful in acute painful exacerbations of chronic ischaemia, especially where surgical or endovascular revascularization is not feasible, for example, iloprost, GTN, alcohol, papaverine, and reserpine. In the treatment of thromboangiitis obliterans (TAO), long-term anticoagulants and adrenocortical steroids are also used with little evidence base. However, due to the multiple levels of involvement this condition is not amenable to surgical bypass treatment.

### 18.4.2  Analgesic therapy

Analgesic therapy is not aimed at improving ischaemia but at reducing pain. Non-opioid analgesics such as paracetamol and non-steroidal non-inflammatory drugs can be useful in mild pain, but frequently opioid-based analgesics are necessary.

Strong opioids such as morphine and fentanyl are indicated in severe ischaemic pain. When patients are unable to eat or drink, an intravenous patient-controlled analgesia device is best at providing individual levels of pain relief. A number of patients present with vascular occlusive disease related to a history of drug misuse. These patients may need escalating doses of opioids and involvement of the drug dependency unit is essential.

### 18.4.3  Analgesic adjuncts

Pain from ischaemic nerves and arterial ulcers can give rise to complex regional pain syndrome with severe neuropathic pain.

Antidepressants such as amitriptyline and SSRIs have been used with mixed results. Anticonvulsants such as gabapentin and pregabalin are indicated in neuropathic pain particularly after limb amputation.

Systemic lidocaine, a sodium channel blocker, reduces neuropathic pain.

Specific regional blocks

- Regional chemical sympathectomy
- Cervicothoracic (stellate) ganglion (CTG) block—upper limbs
- Lumbar sympathetic block—lower limbs
- Surgical endoscopic thoracic sympathectomy.

These relieve the ischaemic vasospasm pain, which promotes ulcer healing and reduces the incidence of gangrene. This is effective in relieving ischaemic pain at rest (small vessel disease), and in a small proportion it helps with intermittent claudication (medium size vessels). However, it remains unclear whether sympathetic blockade improves the muscular perfusion. Also, the procedure is not without risk, and should be preceded by several diagnostic/prognostic blocks before permanent neurodestructive lesioning is performed. The pain relief is not consistent and relapses are common.

### 18.4.4 Cervicothoracic (stellate) ganglion block

#### 18.4.4.1 *Anatomy*

The cervical sympathetic trunk comprises three ganglia: superior, middle, and inferior ganglia. In 80% of the population, the lowest cervical ganglia is fused with the upper thoracic ganglion to form the CTG. The CTG lies on/lateral to the longus colli muscle at the base of the seventh transverse process and the neck of the first rib. The CTG receives preganglionic fibres from the spinal cord lateral grey column. The preganglionic fibres of the head and neck emerge from the upper five thoracic segment between T2 and T6, which also synapses in the CTG. Approximately 30% of the postganglionic sympathetic supply to the upper limb passes directly out of the thoracic outlet from the T2–T8 fibres to the brachial plexus and thus escapes the stellate ganglion (fused C7–T1 ganglia). Thus, the presence of the Horner syndrome (ipsilateral partial ptosis, myosis, enophthalmos, anhydrosis, nasal congestion) does not guarantee complete sympatholysis of the upper limb.

The duration of relief is variable, but with repeated blocks the overall level of sympathetic-mediated pain may be reduced. Destructive lesioning, for example, radiofrequency ablation, is avoided to prevent a permanent Horner syndrome.

#### 18.4.4.2 *Technique*

The block can be performed using anatomical landmarks or by using fluoroscopy. The latter has the advantage of visualization of the C7 transverse process (which if targeted carries a higher risk of pneumothorax and intra-arterial injection) and visualization of the local anaesthetic spread. Intravenous access is mandatory, as the procedure is associated with rare but significant complications.

The patient is supine with a small pillow placed between the shoulders to improve neck extension. The patient is asked to keep their mouth open to relax the neck muscles, avoid speaking/coughing, instead communicate by squeezing the hand of the assistant.

After palpation of the cricoid cartilage, the surface landmark of the C6 transverse process, the carotid pulse is palpated and the carotid sheath is displaced laterally. A 22-gauge, short-beveled needle is attached via a three way tap with a short extension to the 8–12mL local anaesthetic solution syringe (fixed remote technique). The needle is advanced between the sternocleidomastoid and the trachea until bone is encountered (C6 Chassaignac's tubercle). The needle is then withdrawn 3–5mm to avoid injection into longus colli muscle. Negative aspiration is confirmed and a test dose of 0.5mL is injected to exclude intravascular injection, since this could result in seizure and unconsciousness. This is then followed by 8–12mL of the local anaesthetic solution (the concentration can be reduced as the autonomic C-fibres are small and unmyelinated).

### 18.4.4.3 *Complications*

- Horner's syndrome
- Seizures, unconsciousness
- Hoarseness, due to block of recurrent laryngeal nerve
- Phrenic nerve block
- Air embolism
- Pneumothorax
- Infection and haematoma.

### 18.4.5 **Lumbar sympathetic block—lower limbs**

#### 18.4.5.1 *Anatomy*

The psoas major muscle and fascia separate the sympathetic chain from the somatic nerves between L2 and L5. The lumbar sympathetic chain contain both preganglionic and postganglionic fibres to the pelvis and lower limbs. The sympathetic chain and ganglia are closely situated to the anterolateral side of vertebral bodies at the lumbar level; ideal needle placement between lower third L2 to upper third L3 body. The rami communicantes runs as a tortuous tunnel around the vertebral body. Hence, the risk with the paramedian approach for a neurolytic sympathectomy is that the neurolytic agent could backtrack causing a painful somatic neuritis.

#### 18.4.5.2 *Technique*

Fluoroscopy is used to confirm needle placement. Temperature probes attached to the patent's feet can monitor skin temperature. The patient's back is prepared and draped. Local anaesthetic is injected 7–10cm lateral to L3 spinous process. A 22-gauge 20cm needle is directed to upper third of L3; with loss of resistance felt when needle tip is anterior to the psoas fascia. Injected contrast shows a linear spread along anterolateral aspect of vertebral body. Then inject 15–20mL of local anaesthetic (e.g., 0.375% bupivacaine) while monitoring the increase in the ipsilateral foot temperature.

During a neurolytic block, a solution of 6% phenol with radio-opaque contrast (e.g., Conray-420 dye) is used, to aid visibility. The injection is performed with the radiographic C-arm in the lateral position to detect any retrograde spread of the dye, with resultant somatic neuritis.

### 18.4.5.3 *Complications*

- Bleeding, perforation of lumbar vessels, aorta
- Orthostatic hypotension
- Perforation of abdominal viscera
- Subarachnoid or epidural injection
- Backache and muscle spasm
- Nerve root injury
- Haematuria.

## 18.5 **Phantom limb (post-amputation) pain**

Phantom limb pain is very distressing and almost all amputees suffer from phantom limb pain at some stage. The non-existent limb is painful commonly of shooting and burning nature. There is some evidence that severe preamputation pain can result in an increase in the post-operative phantom limb pain.

Patient can describe phantom sensations, which are not painful and to treat these is questionable. Stump pain should alert the clinician to look for an underlying cause such as neuroma or infection. Ongoing infection can exacerbate phantom limb pain.

The pain arising from tissue disruption and nerve transection leads to

- Stress and anxiety induced sympathetically enhanced circulation in the remaining limb's disrupted circulatory bed
- Central nervous system plasticity due to neuronal growth
- Hypersensitivity of the receptive fields adjoining the amputation site
- Ectopically initiated signals from newly cut nerves, sensitized by the cascades of inflammatory mediators released from local tissue trauma
- Spasms of the muscles no longer attached to their origins
- Changes in circulatory pressure balances due to the amount of tissue removed
- Decreased perfusion to the distal end of the residual limb due to disruption of the net capillary return.

### 18.5.1 **Management of phantom limb pain**

#### 18.5.1.1 *Epidural*

Pre-emptive (24hr) preoperative epidural and continuous infusion 3 days post-operatively (combined with perineural local anaesthesia) has been shown to reduce residual limb pain and phantom pain up to 12 months post-operation.

Techniques to improve placement (from the interlaminar or caudal approach) include

• Fluoroscopy with injected contrast
• Ultrasound
• Continuous electrographic monitoring via a specially devised catheter (Tsui test).

#### 18.5.1.2 *Complications*

• Infection, epidural abscess
• Bleeding, epidural haematoma
• Backache
• Vasovagal, cardiovascular collapse
• Neurological complications: aseptic meningitis, paraplegia, quadriplegia, arachnoiditis
• Post-dural puncture headache
• Systemic complications related to corticosteroid and local anaesthetic injection.

Epidural analgesia is limited and pain often persists long after discontinuation and can be severe. It is important to address phantom limb pain as soon as it arises and pain assessment should always include question regarding stump pain, phantom sensation, and most importantly phantom limb pain. Strong opioids are indicated and together with neuropathic agents can control symptoms. There is little evidence in the literature how long to continue such therapy, however, one best follows the patient's progress. Short-term adjuncts to conventional treatments in phantom limb pain include TENS, hypnosis, and acupuncture, however, with mixed response rates.

In intractable pain, invasive treatments, such as dorsal route entry zone lesions and dorsal spinal cord stimulation, have been shown to be successful in case reports.

The health care teams must balance the need for effective analgesia and the patient's ability to comply with rehabilitation; as rapid ambulation and use of residual limb is crucial to recovery. Clinical psychologists on the health care team provide preoperative education about the sensations the patient should expect post-operation and the rehabilitation process. This includes education on patience, stress control, relaxation training, and to understand that phantom sensation are normal and expected. Later, they can provide psychological cognitive behavioural therapy.

# References

Cambou JP, Aboyans V, Constans J, Lacroix P, Dentans C, Bura A (2010). Characteristics and outcome of patients hospitalised for lower extremity peripheral artery disease in France: The Copart Registry. *Eur J Endovasc Surg*, **18**.

Gofeld M, Bhatia A, Abbas S, Ganapathy S, Johnson M (2009). Development and validation of a new technique for ultrasound-guided stellate ganglion block. *Reg Anesth Pain Med*, **34**(5), 475–9.

Halbert J, Crotty M, Cameron ID (2002). Evidence for the optimal management of acute and chronic phantom pain: a systematic review. *Clin J Pain*, **18**(2), 84–92.

Jensen TS, Nikolajsen L (2000). Pre-emptive analgesia in postamputation pain: an update. *Prog Brain Res*, **129**, 493–503.

# Index

185

## H

## I

## J

# P